Carpal Tunnel Syndrome
and Repetitive Strain Injuries

Carpal Tunnel Syndrome and Repetitive Strain Injuries

The Comprehensive Guide to Prevention, Treatment and Recovery

by Tammy Crouch

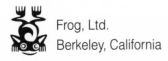

Frog, Ltd.
Berkeley, California

This book is dedicated to my dad,
William A. Scraper
May 5, 1913–April 13, 1995

Carpal Tunnel Syndrome and Repetitive Strain Injuries

Copyright © 1995 Tammy Crouch. No portion of this book, except for brief review, may be reproduced in any form without written permission of the publisher. For information contact Frog, Ltd. c/o North Atlantic Books.

Published by Frog, Ltd.

Frog, Ltd. books are distributed by
North Atlantic Books
P.O. Box 12327
Berkeley, CA 94712

Cover photograph by Richard Blair
Cover and book design by Leigh McLellan

Printed in the United States of America

Library of Congress Cataloging-in-Publication Data

Crouch, Tammy.
      Carpal tunnel syndrome and repetitive stress injuries :
   the comprehensive guide to prevention, treatment, and
   recovery / by Tammy Crouch.
            p.   m.
      Includes bibliographical references and index.
      ISBN 1-883319-50-1 (pbk.)
      1. Carpal Tunnel Syndrome. 2. Overuse injuries. I. Title.
RC422.C26C764   1966
616.8'7—dc20   96-8576
                                                        CIP

1 2 3 4 5 6 7 8 9 / 99 98 97 96 95

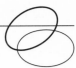

Contents

CHAPTER SIX   **Stress Management**   65

CHAPTER SEVEN   **Prevention and Self-Help**   77

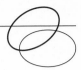

Acknowledgments

I could not have completed this book without the generous support and assistance of the many people around the country who took the time to respond to my questionnaires, answer my many questions over the phone, send me books, articles, and videos, or agree to meet with me in person. Many times someone would call me for information and end up being interviewed for this book. To all of you, my deepest appreciation.

Special thanks to the following for their professional advice:

Dr. Paul Kratka ("The Carpal Tunnel Doctor")—Your dedication, encouragement and enthusiasm were a great inspiration to me. Many, many thanks.

Ray C. Wunderlich, Jr., M.D.—for your generosity in allowing me to refer to your excellent booklet on CTS, your kind letters, and for your open mind . . . thank you!

Dr. Dena Lendrum—your professionalism, skill, humor, and openness to new ideas continue to restore my faith in the medical community during my sometimes frustrating search for answers, whether to my own physical challenges or those of the world. Thanks for taking such good care of me and my family, and for always looking for zebras.

Also:

All my friends and colleagues on Prodigy, America Online, Delphi, SOREHAND, RSI Newsletter, and throughout the Internet for providing me with so much information and support. Together we'll put an end to the "Inflammation Superhighway"!

Jackie Ross, Gary Karp, Dr. Linda Haack-Rogers, Robin Coutellier, Dan Wallach, Colleen Timmons, Dr. William Previte, Dr. Robert Gelb, Dr. John Ford, Greg Bilg, William Mann, Lisa Williams, and Michael Krugman, along with Kathy Glass, and Lindy Hough and Richard Grossinger of North Atlantic Books.

Models for the photographs in the book are: Cheance Adair, Rob Balaam, Lalyn Bellman, John Crouch, Kristie Hickok, Michael Madden, Liz Mendoza, Michael Sullivan.

Personal thanks to:

Cheance Adair, for your help with photos, graphics, surveys, promotion, parking meter money, and all the other millions of things you do that I never thank you for enough,

Michael Madden, D.C., thanks to you, Jim, Vickie, and the dolphins for assistance in the original project and continuing encouragement, support, medical references, and humor.

Erin Melissa Crouch, for grounding me and making me laugh when I've been at the computer too long (who needs "Lifeguard" when you've got a five-year-old?),

And, as always, to my husband, John Crouch, all my thanks for everything you do to keep me going, including typing when my hands wore out, mailing out innumerable questionnaires, weathering a storm or two, and keeping a smile on my face.

Tammy Crouch
March 10, 1996

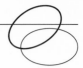

Introduction

My first book on Carpal Tunnel Syndrome and overuse injuries[1] was written as a sort of catharsis for my own sometimes frustrating experiences as a patient. There was simply no unbiased source of information on current treatment options, diagnostic tests, exercises, or ideas for self-help and prevention at the time I was diagnosed with CTS in 1984. So, for the next eight years, I became as educated as I could about the causes and cures of overuse injuries.

My motivation at first was purely selfish—I wanted full use of my hands again. As my own symptoms began to improve, my interest expanded to include my co-workers, some thirty-odd sign language interpreters and instructors whose injury rate at the time was nearly 90%. When I shared what I knew with them, and more importantly, our administrators (who shared our concerns and supported us wholeheartedly), people slowly started getting better. Injury reports decreased. We began working with employees, teaching exercises and self-help techniques. And after years of lectures, seminars, one-on-one training, and the accumulation of a small mountain of

---

1. *Carpal Tunnel Syndrome and Overuse Injuries: Prevention, Treatment, and Recovery* (North Atlantic Books, 1992).

handouts, articles, and product information, I finally sat down and wrote the book I wish I'd had when *my* symptoms first began. I knew that there was a need in my own community for this information, but nothing could have prepared me for the reception the book received nationwide. Patients wrote and called, sharing their own stories. I heard from health care professionals, happy to share the most current information from their particular specialties or occasionally to grouse about a treatment I'd included that they didn't like. I soon found myself passing out new, expanded surveys (2,000 this time!) and collecting a whole new batch of information. For the many people all over the country who were anxious to share their experiences, for the health care professionals who wanted to help by telling me what they do and how it works—this book is for you. I've enjoyed putting it together in the hopes it can answer questions for some of you, and raise questions for others.

This book won't tell you what to do for your particular case of aching hands and sore wrists. I don't have a program to sell or a technique to promote that will cure everyone's ills (and if someone you know claims to, run!), nor am I a health care practitioner or someone who earns a living from treating repetitive strain injuries. I was a patient, like most of you, and what I set out to do was to gather as much information as I could on a variety of different treatment philosophies, self-help ideas, and resources, in the hopes that those of you looking for answers could find a starting point here. You'll find contradictions and disagreements between patients and practitioners, because that's the way it is in real life. You'll read about patients who improved dramatically with a particular treatment, and others who became worse from an identical procedure. That's the reality; we're all different, with different bodies, habits, job duties, diets, and other health factors. What you *will* find here are options—ideas that I hope will help you in your search for your own individual treatment plan. And while I believe strongly in the value of self-help techniques and home care, I've included information on dealing with the real world of RSIs, including doctors, employers, and everything you need to know to be an informed consumer of medical services.

After more than twelve years of living with and researching these disorders, I can tell you the one and only singula1r thing which is needed by *every* repetitive strain injury patient is this: ***education***. I've tried to make this book as unbiased and comprehensive as possible. Your feedback is always welcome, and I can be reached through my publisher by writing to:

North Atlantic Books
1456 Fourth Street
Berkeley, California 94710

I am currently in the process of designing a Repetitive Strain Injury Home Page on the World Wide Web. For now, I can be reached electronically at:

tmcrouch@aol.com.

Although we all know health care professionals may be male *or* female, the use of s/he and him/her is awkward. Thus, throughout the book I have varied the gender when referring to care providers.

This book is in no way intended as a substitute for the care of a professional health practitioner. If you suspect you may be suffering from any of the conditions discussed herein, *see your physician without delay,* and check with your doctor before trying any of the ideas presented here.

Tammy Crouch talks about Carpal Tunnel Syndrome on the Internet at
http://members.aol.com/tmcrouch/ris/rsi.html

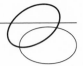

CHAPTER ONE

The Basics

If experiencing the symptoms and limitations of Carpal Tunnel Syndrome is not alarming enough, being confronted with the myriad of choices, opinions, and decisions related to medical care can seem overwhelming. Which treatment is best for me? How can I keep the situation from getting worse? What *is* Carpal Tunnel Syndrome? In just a few short years we've gone from a time when very few people had even heard of Carpal Tunnel Syndrome and repetitive strain injuries to being bombarded on a daily basis with advertisements for ergonomic furniture, hair brushes, even ergonomically designed *homes!* Go out shopping today wearing a wrist splint and chances are you'll have a dozen encounters with complete strangers who'll want to tell you about *their* aching wrists and tingling fingers. And you'll find no shortage of advice about what you should do to get well. The truth is, obtaining an accurate diagnosis and then finding the proper treatment for your individual case is often a complicated and time-consuming process.

An important first step in making the right choices as a patient is understanding how your body works. Some basic information about anatomy can help you keep track of your symptoms and understand your treatment. There is no substitute for the services of a qualified health care professional, and under no circumstances do I encourage you to diagnose or treat your-self. However, having some basic knowledge to call upon not only gives you a better chance of recovery, but helps you act as a full-fledged member of your own health care team.

Nerves and How They Work

The human nervous system is nothing short of miraculous. As you read this sentence, nerve cells all over your body are receiving and transmitting im-pulses to and from your brain, your glands, your internal and sensory or-gans, your skin, all the billions of functioning parts of you—and mostly without your conscious awareness.

When you wiggle your fingers, a message is dispatched from your brain to your digits, commanding them to move. When you touch a hot pan, a sensory impulse ("pain!") enters your central nervous system, causing you to immediately withdraw the hand and perhaps even to vocalize with an exclamation suitable for the occasion.

When an injury or illness disrupts that flow of information between the nerves and the brain or vice versa, problems ensue. Carpal Tunnel Syndrome is the name of one condition affecting the nerves of the hand, specifically the *median nerve.*

The bones (or vertebrae) that make up your spine are separated by disks made of a gelatinous cartilage surrounded by an outer ring, the annulus fibrosus. These disks cushion the vertebrae during movement, absorb the shock caused by walking, running and jumping, permit the spinal column to bend and twist, and prevent damage to the spinal nerves, which enter and exit the spinal cord through openings in the vertebrae. There are thirty-one pairs of spinal nerves, originating in the spinal cord and following their own particular routes throughout the body. The median nerve starts in the neck from the area of the seventh and eighth vertebrae, and runs all the way down to the hand, carrying signals between the hand and the brain. The median nerve performs two functions: *sensory*—it allows the hand to feel sensations and relays them to the central nervous system, and *motor*—the median nerve receives messages from the brain and allows the hand to move and do things.

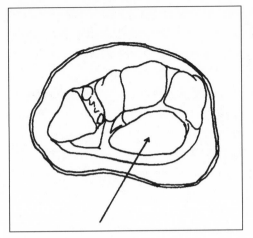

Figure 1. The carpal tunnel

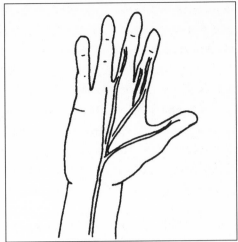

Figure 2. The median nerve

The Carpal Tunnel

The *carpal tunnel* is a narrow space in the wrist [Figure 1]. Three walls of the "tunnel" are made up of the eight carpal bones, while the fourth is formed by the tough transverse carpal ligament, or *flexor retinaculum,* Through the tunnel pass nine *tendons,* tough bands of connective tissue that attach the muscles of the arm to the bones in the hand. These tendons are the four profundus tendons, the four superficialis tendons, and the flexor pollicis longus tendon.

Nerves that carry messages between the brain and the hand also pass through the narrow carpal tunnel. The median nerve is shown in Figure 2.

Carpal Tunnel Syndrome

Carpal Tunnel Syndrome has been known by many names—repetitive strain injury, cumulative trauma disorder, occupational neuritis, and others. As long ago as 1854 Sir James Paget described a condition involving chronic compression of the median nerve at the wrist. In 1947 Dr. George Phalen made his first diagnosis of Carpal Tunnel Syndrome. Estimates of people affected by Carpal Tunnel Syndrome range from one percent of the general population to as high as *thirty-five percent* of those whose hobbies or work involve repetitive wrist and hand movements. It is no wonder that CTS is the subject of extensive research and attention from all facets of the medical community.

Many factors can cause pressure on the median nerve. If for any reason the contents of the carpal tunnel become larger or swollen, due to inflammation, for example, or the tunnel itself becomes smaller, the median nerve can become pinched or irritated. Inflammation and swelling around the tendons and nerve can lead to a variety of sensory and motor symptoms which are collectively known as ***Carpal Tunnel Syndrome.*** These symptoms include:

Sensory	**Motor**
numbness, especially at night	loss of hand strength
tingling	weakness of thumb
burning	smaller thumb muscles
coldness	clumsiness, dropping things
pain and/or stiffness	problems grasping or pinching

Symptoms may be felt in the hand (especially the thumb, index, and middle fingers), wrist, up into the elbow, and even in the shoulder. Often these feelings are worse at night, and the pain and tingling can be severe enough to wake a person from a sound sleep. In the early stages, patients

---

"It's like a feeling of pins and needles."

"Feels as if my hand is asleep."

"I have shooting pains down my forearm."

"My handwriting became illegible."

"Feels like I just hit my 'funny bone'."

" I began dropping things . . . my grip became weak."

"Both hands and wrists became swollen."

"At night my hands would fall asleep from wrist to fingertips and ache!"

often try to get temporary relief by shaking the hand out or massaging the area. In most cases, however, consistent use of the hand will gradually increase the symptoms, and as the problem becomes worse the motor portion of the nerve is involved. This affects the ability to use the hand. It becomes more difficult to perform small, specific tasks such as buttoning clothes and picking up small items, and hand strength is often affected.

A variety of factors can contribute to the development of Carpal Tunnel Syndrome or its symptoms, from an injury to the wrist area to a problem with general health. Only you and your health care professional can determine the cause of your symptoms. A thorough medical examination is vital when experiencing symptoms like those described here. *Do not try to diagnose yourself.* I've heard from people who've been "diagnosed" by friends, co-workers, even over electronic mail on a computer bulletin board! Be sure what you have is, in fact, Carpal Tunnel Syndrome, and find out what physical and/or environmental factors played a part in its development.

"There's No Such Thing!"

You may have encountered by now the skeptics out there—be they disgruntled employers, overworked spouses, or even well-meaning friends who just can't see anything wrong with you. One physician insisted to me that Carpal Tunnel Syndrome was nothing more than an elaborate insurance scam, a bandwagon full of hypochondriacs and malingerers bent on taking a bite out of some poor Workers' Compensation insurance company. The fact that it seems to affect more women than men doesn't help the situation. Is there such a thing as Carpal Tunnel Syndrome?

YES—at least according to the majority of health care professionals. Compression or irritation of the median nerve at the wrist can generally be verified through a variety of orthopedic and especially *neurological* diagnostic tests. Are these tests always performed on every patient with wrist pain or numbness in the fingers? No, unfortunately they are not. In some cases, the diagnosis of Carpal Tunnel Syndrome is either incomplete or incorrect. Adding to the arsenal of the skeptics are the folks who see feigning a wrist injury as a ticket to some time off with pay from an unhappy work situation. The legitimate cases of Carpal Tunnel Syndrome far outnumber the

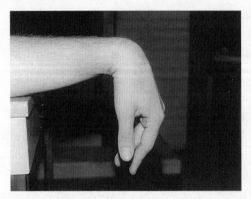
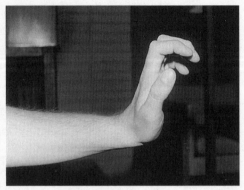

Figure 3. Hyperflexion   Figure 4. Hyperextension

fraudulent claims, but to imagine that a small percentage of malingerers doesn't exist is wishful thinking. I've seen them, and they make it doubly hard for those with genuine injuries to be taken seriously.

Carpal Tunnel Syndrome exists. But is the term sometimes overused or misunderstood? Definitely.

Repetitive Strain Injuries

One cause of Carpal Tunnel Syndrome is known as cumulative trauma. When the hand is used repeatedly over long periods of time, the muscles and tendons become susceptible to microscopic tearing and fatigue. Without sufficient rest and time to heal, chronic *inflammation* results. Inflammation is the body's natural response to injury. The increased blood flow and fluid to the area may show up as redness, heat, or swelling, and the inflamed nerve endings cause pain. Pain is your body's way of telling you to take it easy, to allow tissue repair to begin. Ignoring the signals your body is sending you may lead to a worsening of the problem.

Excessive amounts of *hyperflexion* and/or *hyperextension* [see Figures 3 and 4] can cause the joints and tendons of the wrist to become inflamed and swollen, in turn compressing the median nerve. Remember, the carpal tunnel is a very small, inelastic space, housing nine tendons plus the median nerve. If the contents of the carpal tunnel become larger due to swelling or inflam-

Another Theory

SOREHAND, an international computerized "discussion" group concerned with repetitive stress injuries like Carpal Tunnel Syndrome, shared this information as an alternative to the theory of swelling or inflammation within the carpal tunnel as the cause of CTS: "Dr. Hunter in 'Recurrent Carpal Tunnel Syndrome. . .,' Hand Clinics 7:3 pp. 491–504, says that there is actually 'plenty of room' in the carpal tunnel under most circumstances. In particular, for tendon surgery he sometimes places up to 4 rods into the carpal tunnel, and these additions almost never lead to Carpal Tunnel Syndrome. He has evidence that Carpal Tunnel Syndrome may more often relate to adhesions leading to tension/traction on the nerve than to compression in the tunnel as is often supposed."

mation, there is simply no extra room in the already crowded tunnel, and pressure on the median nerve results. That pressure can lead to changes in the sensory and motor aspects of the hand.

"Why Do My Symptoms Seem Worse at Night?"

One explanation for this common pattern is that blood flows through your system much slower at night, which can enlarge the blood vessels at the carpal tunnel. The increased amount of blood puts pressure on the nerve. This may account for the increased numbness, tingling, and pain some people experience at night.

Also, the position of your hands and arms as you sleep can play a major part in worsening symptoms of CTS. If you sleep with your hands in a hyperflexed or hyperextended position you may very well wake up with hands that feel as if they are "asleep." Changing habits that occur while you sleep is difficult, but it can be done. Many CTS patients find that wearing wrist splints to bed keeps the hands in a more neutral position and relieves some of the pressure on the median nerve.

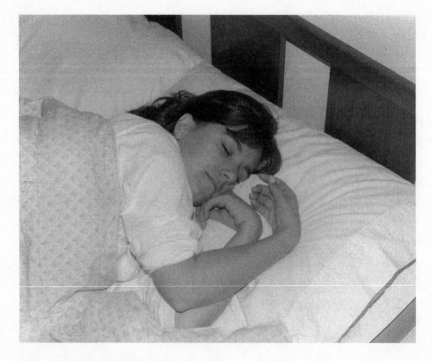

Figure 5. Sleeping positions like this can worsen symptoms.

Who Gets Carpal Tunnel Syndrome?

In 1994 the Bureau of Labor Statistics reported that about 339,000 occupational injuries involved repetitive stress disorders in the upper extremities.[2] The Bureau documented 302,000 RSIs in 1993, and 281,000 in 1992. These injuries are the fastest growing, most widespread occupational hazard in today's workplace. The majority of people diagnosed with CTS carry out with some kind of repetitive task in the workplace or home involving the use of hands or fingers. The application of force, pressure from hard work surfaces, vibration and certain hand tools have all been shown to increase the incidence of CTS. Repeated pressure in the joint as well as the increased size of muscles and tendons pressing on the median nerve in the wrist all serve to exacerbate the problem.

---

2. Time Magazine, June 1995.

- computer operators
- retail clerks
- food servers
- assembly workers
- musicians

- hairstylists
- typists
- sign language interpreters
- construction workers
- butchers

Not only do people in the above occupations use their hands a lot, but many of them also must bend the neck or look down in order to perform the required duties of their jobs. In upcoming chapters you'll learn why this creates an even greater likelihood for the development of repetitive strain injury.

"Why Me?"

"I work in a legal office with four other secretaries. We all do the same amount of typing, but I'm the only one experiencing CTS. Why me?"

There's no definitive answer for the question of why some of us end up with aching hands while others perform the same activities pain-free. There are many theories—vitamin deficiencies, wrist shape (see below), condition of the neck and spine, posture, overall health and physical condition, and work habits, to name a few. Perhaps it is as simple as the individual's particular response to physical or even emotional stresses. Just as some people don't succumb to this year's flu virus, some employees who use their hands in a repetitive fashion don't end up with CTS. And some people who don't really use their hands excessively at all end up in splints. There's no hard and fast rule to determine which individuals will experience overuse injuries. One orthopedic surgeon (a man I came across regularly doling out "professional" diagnoses—which nearly always included a recommendation for surgery—over a computer service, and who, interestingly, refused to be interviewed for this book) I corresponded with stated emphatically, "There's no such thing as a repetitive stress injury. Either you're going to get it or you're not, and there's nothing you can do to prevent it. Calling CTS a work-related injury is just another way to take advantage of the Workers' Compensation system." This point of view may seem a bit extreme, but it is one of the many ways people view the issue.

Wrist Shape and Carpal Tunnel Syndrome

Could the shape of your wrist indicate your likelihood of developing Carpal Tunnel Syndrome? It's a factor worth considering, says San Diego chiropractor Dr. Michael Madden. "A three-year study at Ohio State University found three times greater evidence of nerve damage in autoworkers with 'square' wrists as compared to those with 'rectangular' ones. A 'square' wrist was defined as one that was almost as thick as it was wide. The doctors involved in the study speculated that the way the tendons lay in the 'square' wrist may cause greater pressure on the nerve. How can you determine your own wrist shape? Using a caliper from a medical or art supply store, measure both the height and width at the crease closest to the palm. Divide the thickness measurement by the width. A ratio of 0.7 or higher indicates a 'square' wrist and possible increased risk for CTS."[3] Can wrist shape increase your chances of developing Carpal Tunnel Syndrome? Clearly, more research is needed before a connection can be considered definite. However, it is true that while many employees in a particular office may perform nearly identical functions, only *some* of them will develop CTS. Why? Wrist shape may indeed be one of many factors, including posture, workstation design, and overall health and physical condition.

Stages I, II, and III

In my initial work with Dr. Madden on the prevention and treatment of Carpal Tunnel Syndrome, we found it helpful to divide the stages of CTS into three categories: *Stage I*—mild symptoms with negative test results; *Stage II*—moderate symptoms with positive results from orthopedic and/or neurological testing; and *Stage III*—moderate to severe symptoms with significant abnormalities on the electromyographic studies.

---

3. Published in the *American Journal of Physical Medicine and Rehabilitation*, date unknown.

Stage I

At this early stage, symptoms are mild and tests for damage to the nerve are negative. You may be feeling some intermittent numbness or tingling, and perhaps pain in the wrist or forearm. Usually, a short rest period, a massage, or a session with the chiropractor, physical therapist, or acupuncturist brings relief that lasts for weeks. With a few changes in work habits and lifestyle, chances for a complete recovery are excellent. If you are just beginning to experience the symptoms of repetitive stress injury, take the opportunity to scrutinize your workstation, habits, stress level, and diet. Your body is trying to tell you something. Many times with a little detective work you will be able to identify some of the factors that contribute to your symptoms. Now, change the things you can—make protecting your hands a priority, and your prospects for never seeing Stage II or III are good.

What Do Health Care Practitioners Recommend?

I asked a wide variety of health care professionals the following question: "What do you suggest for the initial stage of Carpal Tunnel Syndrome?"

Some of their responses include:

- "Soft tissue manipulation of the head and shoulders, and acupuncture."
- "Splint at night."
- "I request that the client take rest from whatever action is causing the dysfunction. Massage [directed to] forearm, hand and shoulder. I also look for deeper organic imbalance."
- "Vitamin C and B6."
- "Activity modification, wrist splint, vitamin B6."
- "Splint and anti-inflammatory medication."

Each case is different. See your own doctor for recommendations specific to your particular condition.

Stage II

In Stage II Carpal Tunnel Syndrome, symptoms are moderate and orthopedic and neurological tests are *positive*. With your health care provider's approval, the suggestions for self-help, home care, and professional therapy should be continued at this point—they may bring a great deal of relief and prevent the injury from worsening.

When diagnostic tests, particularly neurological studies, are positive, there is damage to the nerve requiring a somewhat more aggressive approach. Taking a ten-minute break may not be enough any more. Patients with Stage II CTS often report that symptoms like pain and tingling continue for some time even after the aggravating activity is stopped. Obtaining relief takes a longer rest period, extended periods wearing a splint or forearm brace, or more frequent visits to the doctor for therapy.

Depending on the amount of nerve damage, the success of the treatment program, and the patient's ability to make changes in habits and lifestyle, Stage II CTS patients can either achieve a full or partial recovery or the condition can worsen into Stage III Carpal Tunnel Syndrome.

Stage III

When patients have moderate to severe symptoms for more than one year or have consistent weakness and/or atrophy of muscles in the thumb, and electromyographic tests (see Chapter Three) show significant abnormalities, they have reached **Stage III** Carpal Tunnel Syndrome.

At this point, there is significant damage to the median nerve and it is difficult to relieve symptoms with any kind of conservative treatment (ice, splints, massage). Patients in Stage III generally experience nearly constant pain in the wrist and hand, and/or numbness and tingling in the fingers. Grip strength can be affected, and the patient may have trouble picking up or holding things. When the thumb and index finger of the injured hand are pinched together, they can be separated easily due to weakness of the muscles. The muscle at the base of the thumb may actually begin to shrink in size or *atrophy,* or actually waste away. At this point, there is no question that some kind of medical intervention is necessary to prevent further, and possibly irreparable, nerve damage.

Some doctors may fashion a device that goes beyond the immobilization of the wrist splint—a sort of removable cast that is worn everywhere
except the shower or bath. This can be helpful when total immobilization is
necessary to allow the injured limb to rest. Carpal Tunnel Syndrome patients can attest to the difficulty of not using the hands—it's nearly impossible. But in Stage III Carpal Tunnel Syndrome, it is advisable to completely
discontinue any activity that will worsen the injury. The nerve needs a
chance to heal, and it can't without rest. Your physician can help you determine the length of time needed for complete rest.

If damage to the nerve has progressed to the point where more conservative methods fail, your physician may suggest surgery as soon as possible
to release the entrapped nerve and prevent further damage. In Chapter Five
I discuss surgery in detail.

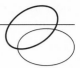

CHAPTER TWO

Horses And Zebras
or "If It Isn't Carpal Tunnel Syndrome, What *Is* It?"

It is a common misconception that if you have symptoms such as tingling and numbness in the hands and fingers, the cause of the symptoms *must* be found there, too. "When you hear hoofbeats," I've heard again and again, "look for horses, not zebras!" However, when Carpal Tunnel Syndrome is suspected, a good health care professional will look for horses, zebras, and *wildebeests* if necessary for a thorough and accurate diagnosis. Anything less is substandard medical care. Occasionally, an "official" diagnosis of Carpal Tunnel Syndrome is made just from the patient's history of numbness or tingling in the fingers alone. From what you learned in the first chapter about nerves and how they work, you now know that it isn't always that simple.

There are a number of places along the pathway of the median nerve where inflammation and/or compression can occur, creating a variety of conditions with symptoms which may appear quite similar to Carpal Tunnel Syndrome. In some cases there is nerve irritation or compression, in others the problem relates to muscles, tendons, or ligaments.

Carpal Tunnel Syndrome is not the only injury related to overuse of the hands and arms. The forearm, elbow, and shoulder are also subject to wear and tear from overuse, and there are some specific problems that affect them, as well. Some of the conditions with symptoms similar enough to sometimes be confused with CTS are discussed below.

Conditions Similar to CTS

•   **Spinal Stenosis**   Nerve compression at the spinal column due to a narrowing of the passage through which the nerve passes, which can create symptoms in the hands and wrists.

•   **Disk Herniations**   When all or part of a disk's gelatinous material extrudes through its outer ring, due to trauma, strain, or joint degeneration, it can create pressure on the nerve roots of the spine or even the spinal cord itself. We usually think of herniated disks as occurring in the lower back; however, disk herniations can and do occur in the cervical spine as well, and can create neurologic symptoms similar to those of a repetitive strain injury. Tests to identify a disk herniation include electromyography, magnetic resonance imaging, and neuromuscular tests. Treatment may require bed rest, some kind of supportive brace, neck traction, medications, and, in severe cases, surgery to relieve the pressure. If you have recently had a trauma to the neck, such as a whiplash injury, or suspect a problem with your neck, bring it to your doctor's attention immediately. As with most conditions, early diagnosis and intervention will give you the best chance for a successful recovery.

•   **Thoracic Outlet Compression Syndrome**   Compression occurs where the nerves cross the muscles of the axilla (armpits), shoulders, or ribs. Symptoms of pain and numbness can be felt in the elbow, wrist, or hand.

•   **Cubital Tunnel Syndrome, Ulnar Nerve Impingement Syndrome, Ulnar Neuritis**   These related conditions involve compression or irritation of the ulnar nerve at the elbow. The ulnar nerve is what people often refer to as the "funny bone" [Figure 6] at the elbow. Repetitive trauma can lead to a thickening in this region, usually due to a buildup of scar tissue. The patient feels a tingling sensation in the hand, generally in the fourth and fifth fingers, sometimes accompanied by weakness and pain.

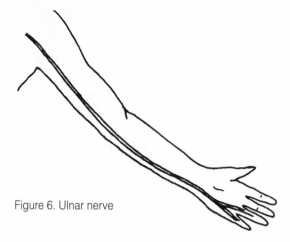

Figure 6. Ulnar nerve

• **Tendinitis** This common ailment results from inflammation of the tendons which, as you recall from Chapter One, are tough fibrous cords that attach muscles to bones. When a tendon is over-stretched, it can become strained, leading to pain and swelling. Injury can occur when the elbow is extended repeatedly, often combined with twisting or flexing the elbow and arm, especially against resistance. And because of the interrelation of the muscles of the elbow and the hands and fingers, overuse of the hands can also cause pain in the elbow, as indicated in Figure 7.

Tendinitis at the elbow is often called "tennis elbow" or "golfer's elbow." There is often a feeling of pain that can spread down the entire length of the

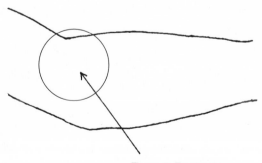

Figure 7. Tendonitus

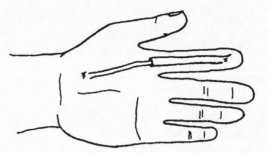

Figure 8. Site of tenosynovitis

forearm as well as up into the shoulder. Grip and general forearm strength are usually affected. Tears in the tendons, muscles, or ligaments will proba-bly feel painful to the touch. Ice and immobilization may be recommended for the initial stages of these injuries, followed by gentle stretching and heat after the inflammation has subsided. The use of a forearm brace can help by partially immobilizing the muscles of the forearm.

•   **Tenosynovitis and DeQuervain's Disease**   Some of the body's tendons are enclosed in a membrane sheath which aids in movement [Figure 8]. Teno-synovitis (sometimes called **"Trigger Finger"**) refers to inflammation of the tendon sheath. An inflamed, tight tendon sheath restricts movement of the tendon.

DeQuervain's Disease, first identified in the nineteenth century by Dr. DeQuervain, a Swiss surgeon, is a form of tenosynovitis which affects a small tunnel along the thumb side of the wrist that transports some exten-sor and thumb tendons. In this disease, there is inflammation which nar-rows the lining of the tunnel, resulting in pain and tenderness around the affected wrist and thumb. Traditional treatment includes immobilization of the thumb and wrist, anti-inflammatory medications, and possibly injec-tions of cortisone. In some cases tenosynovitis can be caused by an infec-tion, in which case treatment with antibiotics may be required.

•   **Reflex Sympathetic Dystrophy**   RSD appears to be related to a mal-function of the sympathetic nervous system, most often occurring after an injury or trauma. Peripheral nerves become hypersensitive, leading to severe burning pain out of proportion to the original injury. RSD often occurs in a limb; however, symptoms can spread beyond the injured site. Other symptoms include skin discoloration, limited range of motion, swelling, increased perspiration, and changes in nail and hair growth. Although there is no standard treatment, physical therapy, nerve-blocking drugs, and splinting to prevent muscle contraction deformities may be beneficial.

- **Ganglion Cysts** Ganglion cysts are small, fluid-filled cysts that can appear on the hands or wrists. Although they are not uncommon, ganglion cysts can become tender and in some cases lead to symptoms of tendinitis in the arm. They are easily removed by your physician, either by aspiration or a minor surgical procedure.

The Neck

Knowing what we do about the cervical spine and its relationship with the route of the nerves that work the hands, it's no wonder that those of us who type hunched over a computer all day, straining our necks to see written materials, may be doubling our chances of developing a repetitive strain injury. One patient from California wrote to me that she had tried everything for her aching hands, including medication and splints, and her doctors were pressuring her to schedule a second surgery (the first one had failed). By accident she found that her symptoms improved dramatically when she purchased a good quality "cervical" pillow—one designed to support her neck in a neutral position while she slept. I've heard dozens of stories from patients who felt relief *in their hands* after neck traction or chiropractic adjustment of the cervical spine.

Adrian R. Upton, M.D., and Alan J. McComas, M.D., from the Department of Medicine at McMaster University Medical Center found in a 1973 study of 115 patients with nerve entrapment at the wrist or elbow that a full seventy percent of them also had nerve irritation at the cervical spine (neck). This is an area of some controversy, but the concept that symptoms in the hand, wrist or fingers could originate at some other point along the nerve is an important consideration when seeking a diagnosis and deciding on treatment.

The "Double Crush Phenomenon"

In some cases, nerve compression can occur at *more than one* point along the nerve's pathway. In 1986 a paper was presented in New Orleans at the 41st annual meeting of the American Society for Surgery of the Hand entitled "Double Crush Syndrome: Cervical Radiculopathy and Carpal Tunnel Syndrome," which set forth the idea that irritation to a nerve anywhere along its pathway will then make other areas of the nerve more susceptible to injury. Dr. Paul Kratka of Carlsbad, California, who specializes in the treatment of Carpal Tunnel Syndrome, discusses how the double crush phenomenon relates to Carpal Tunnel Syndrome in his interview in Chapter Five.

Fibromyalgia Syndrome

Fibromyalgia Syndrome (FMS) is one of those disorders sometimes discounted by the medical world. "Just a fancy word for muscle pain, that's all it is!" Not so for the thousands of people suffering from this potentially disabling condition. Chronic stiffness and pain in the muscles, ligaments, and tendons, along with headaches, fatigue, and non-restorative sleep make Fibromyalgia Syndrome something to be reckoned with for those who have it and their physicians. What causes fibromyalgia is not yet known for sure, and it cannot be confirmed with a particular lab test or x-ray. Most of its sufferers are women. And a substantial number of them have *symptoms* of Carpal Tunnel Syndrome, tendinitis, and other musculoskeletal disorders. In the last ten years or so, medical professionals have developed guidelines that better define FMS, and there is now much more information available on treatment. There is no "cure" for Fibromyalgia Syndrome, but with regular exercise (non-impact, aerobic-type exercise is best—swimming, walking, ski machines), daily stretching, a good diet, plenty of rest, and sometimes medication to control symptoms like inflammation and sleep dysfunction, many patients are able to function well. If you suspect you have FMS, you may visit a rheumatologist, a doctor who specializes in identifying and treating disorders of the joints, muscles, and bones (like arthritis and rheumatism). Or, contact the Arthritis Foundation at 800-283-7800 to request their brochure on Fibromyalgia, or the Fibromyalgia Network at 800-853-2929.

Systemic Disorders

There are other causes of Carpal Tunnel Syndrome or its symptoms that should be ruled out by your physician *before* you attempt the self-help measures described in this book. These include systemic conditions that relate to the whole body, such as:

Diabetes Mellitis	Kidney Dialysis
Hypothyroidism	Use of Oral Contraceptives
Pregnancy	Menopause

Or conditions that affect the actual narrowing of the carpal tunnel, like:

Improperly set fractures or dislocations	Rheumatoid, Osteo and Gouty Arthritis
Pagets Bone Disease	Multiple Myeloma
Acromegaly	Pisiform Hamate Syndrome

As I stress repeatedly in this book, only a qualified health care professional can help you determine the precise cause of your symptoms. Just noticing a connection between typing on the computer and pain in your wrists does not equal an official diagnosis of Carpal Tunnel Syndrome. There could be an underlying physical condition contributing to your symptoms, and *only your doctor* can tell you for sure.

During the last two months of my own pregnancy, both of my hands were completely numb. Within days after delivery, I was back to normal. I've heard from many women who state their symptoms of numbness and pain worsen prior to and during their menstrual periods, probably due to *edema* or fluid retention. Keeping a journal of the ways your symptoms fluctuate will help you detect patterns like these—ways your overall physical condition can affect your hands and arms. In Chapter Seven I share some ideas for keeping a journal.

 Again, if you are experiencing any of the symptoms of Carpal Tunnel Syndrome, please see your doctor without delay.

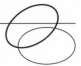

CHAPTER THREE

Obtaining an Accurate Diagnosis

Say you've got a cold. You fight it as best you can for a couple of weeks, but when it's more than you can handle you trundle off to the doctor. Any doctor will do. You're examined, poked, prodded, told you've got strep throat, and sent home with a prescription for an antibiotic. You probably feel much better in a few days. If only identifying and treating a repetitive strain injury were that simple! When Carpal Tunnel Syndrome is the suspected diagnosis, it is impossible to overemphasize the need for a *thorough* physical examination—head to toe, an extensive history, and in many cases an evaluation of the patient's workstation or activities which may have led to the injury.

Regardless of the type of health care practitioner you choose, your examination should include *at least* one of the following diagnostic tests to help determine conclusively whether or not what you are experiencing is Carpal Tunnel Syndrome.

Orthopedic Testing

Orthopedic testing can be a good starting point to detect problems in the wrist and hands. Although a positive or abnormal result cannot be considered

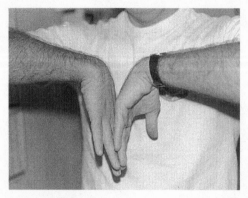

Figure 9. Phalen's test

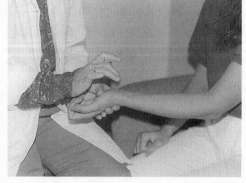

Figure 10. Tinel's test

definitive proof of the existence of Carpal Tunnel Syndrome, it can help you and your doctor decide whether further, more extensive testing is warranted.

The two most common tests to determine problems with the median nerve are the wrist flexion test, or *Phalen's test,* and the median nerve percussion test, or *Tinel's test.*

The wrist flexion test is done by placing the back of the hands together in a bent position, completely flexed, but without force [Figure 9]. If there is any numbness, tingling, or pain within sixty seconds, the test is positive.

Tinel's test is performed by tapping the area over the median nerve on the palm side of the hand [Figure 10]. Again, if tingling or numbness is felt, the test is positive.

Another test used to determine sensitivity in the area is the *Semmes-Weinstein test* [Figure11], where a variety of sizes and weights of plastic rods are touched against the fingertips to test the degree of sensitivity compared to the normal level. This test can sometimes reveal Carpal Tunnel Syndrome symptoms before they become serious, or even before they are noticed by the patient.

The *Vibrometer test* also determines levels of sensitivity through the use of vibration against the fingers. Deviations from the norm can sometimes be present even when the patient has not yet experienced any symptoms.

An instrument called a *Dynamometer* may be used to measure the strength of the patient's grip. The patient squeezes the Dynamometer [Figure12] and the readings are recorded. The dominant hand (usually the one

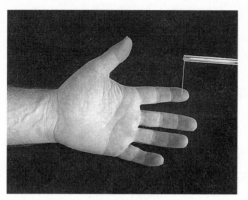

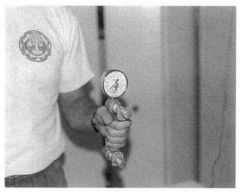

Figure 11. Semmes-Weinstein test   Figure 12. Dynamometer testing

you write with) is generally five to ten pounds stronger than the non-dominant hand—differences from that norm can indicate hand, arm, or even neck involvement.

Doctors may use a variety of objects to test sensitivity along the extremities—a serrated wheel (fondly known by some patients as the "pizza cutter"), a pin, or other object may be dragged lightly across the skin to determine the degree of sensation felt by the patient.

Some health care practitioners employ *applied kinesiology,* a method of muscle testing to discover weaknesses or other neuromuscular problems. Created by chiropractor Dr. George Goodheart, applied kinesiology combines theories of acupuncture and manipulation to measure neurological functioning throughout the body. The practitioner presses on a particular muscle, asks the patient to resist the pressure, and observes the result. To illustrate, your physician may ask you to put out your arm and resist his pressure to push the arm down. You resist the pressure easily. Next, he asks you to keep the arm down as before, but this time as he pushes down on your arm he uses his other hand to simultaneously press down on the top of your head. Boom, the arm goes down with only the slightest pressure, no matter how hard you try to resist the force, and your reaction assists the doctor in determining areas of weakness or dysfunction. Kinesiological testing can also be used to determine the appropriateness of diet and medications. A sugar cube or aspirin on the tongue, for example, or even visualizing an unpleasant event can dramatically affect the body's ability to remain strong.

Applied kinesiology is sometimes employed by doctors of chiropractic medicine who have been trained in this special technique. After making a determination from muscle testing, the practitioner may then decide on a treatment plan of chiropractic adjustments, massage and/or acupressure, nutritional therapy, or specific therapeutic exercises.

X-Rays, Computerized Axial Tomography, and Magnetic Resonance Imaging

Your physician may recommend x-rays of the wrist and arm, or your insurance carrier may require them as part of evaluating your claim. X-rays employ electromagnetic radiation to photograph internal organs and bones. X-rays can be helpful if there has been an actual injury to the wrist—an old fracture, for example, which may not have healed properly. If abnormalities are present, two tests which show a three-dimensional view of the area and the actual size of the carpal tunnel may be helpful. These are the *CAT scan* (also called *CT scan or Computerized Axial Tomography*) or the *MRI (Magnetic Resonance Imaging).* The CAT scan provides three-dimensional, cross-sectional images of various parts of the body, using x-rays but providing far more detail than standard x-rays can. Magnetic Resonance Imaging [Figure 13] uses principles of magnetism to view the contents of the carpal tunnel. Its images are even clearer than those of the CAT scan, and of course the absence of radiation is a plus. Both the CAT scan and the MRI are not only valuable in diagnosing Carpal Tunnel Syndrome, but can be used after treatment to determine progress and response to treatment.

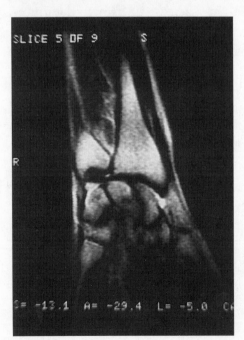

Figure 13. MRI of a hand

Electrodiagnostic Testing

Electrodiagnosis is one of the more reliable methods for identifying abnormalities in the muscles and nerves. Depending on the kind of physician you choose, you may be referred out for this type of testing, or the doctor may perform the tests herself. Special training is required to perform and interpret electrodiagnostic tests. Electrodiagnostic tests may be performed by a *neurologist* (a medical doctor who specializes in nerve disorders) or by a trained technician.

The two most commonly used tests that can help define the "official" presence of Carpal Tunnel Syndrome are the needle *electromyography* (or *EMG*), and nerve conduction studies. The EMG is a test which analyzes the electrical activity in a muscle at rest, upon insertion of a small needle, and during contraction (making a fist, for example). The resulting wave patterns can help the physician identify nerve damage, muscle weakness, and specific muscle diseases, such as myasthenia gravis. Electromyography can be uncomfortable for the patient, particularly when the needle is inserted. Relaxing during the test helps.

Nerve conduction studies involve attaching small electrodes to the skin and then applying an electric stimulus to the nerve. This allows the physician to measure the nerve's response. The impulse may be transmitted at a

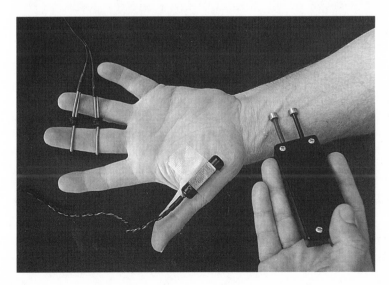

Figure 14. EMG Testing

normal rate, slowly, or not at all, and these findings indicate whether or not there is damage to the nerve (or nearby muscle) and to what extent. Patient tolerance for these tests range from sensing only a mild tingling to a real sense of discomfort. Again, taking some deep breaths and relaxing through the sensations can help immensely, according to technicians and patients I spoke with.

I've had both of the above tests several times, and I found my that perception of the experience varied with my level of muscle tension as well as the practitioner's bedside manner. My first EMG was with a doctor who rushed through the procedure, never stopping to prepare me for what might happen next or how it might feel. And it *hurt.* My second EMG, years later, was performed by a neurologist who took his time, explaining each step along the way, and although his procedure was identical to the first doctor's, the experience for me was quite different. It was still a strange feeling but not at all painful.

With an accuracy rate of ninety percent when the results show abnormalities, electrodiagnostic studies can be a most reliable indicator of any problems with the median and ulnar nerves. However, physical therapist Jackie Ross (see Chapter Five) cautions that false positive findings *can* sometimes occur when muscles of the arm become bound down, compressing the median nerve. Conversely, it is possible to have Carpal Tunnel Syndrome and still have a *negative* (or normal) result from your tests. All the more reason for a comprehensive physical examination along with electrodiagnostic tests.

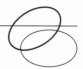

CHAPTER FOUR

Teamwork—
Choosing a Health Care Practitioner

I encourage you to think of yourself as an active participant in your own treatment and recovery process. That attitude shift is essential to a successful treatment program. Our society tends to view doctors as omnipotent, all-knowing, while patients are passive, trusting and uninformed. It is in your best interest to become informed about *any* injury or illness you experience. Don't be afraid to ask questions, read, or talk to others with the same symptoms. Knowledge is your best tool in maintaining your health.

Choosing the Best Doctor for *You*

Selecting the right doctor can be as confusing as trying to pick a needle out of a haystack. The Yellow Pages are full of names of physicians and therapists, some with showy, full-page ads and others with simply a name and address. How do you know which one will give you the best care for your money? Not all doctors or health professionals are familiar with repetitive strain injuries. Sometimes, if the symptoms are not considered severe enough, treatment will be delayed. Physicians have many different philosophies and ways of looking at patients with pain.

Some people choose a particular physician by a referral from their family physician. Doctors may refer their patients to another physician or specialist for a specific problem. And generally speaking, a referral from a doctor you *trust,* who has a thorough understanding of your health and your needs, can be one of the very best ways to find excellent health care. The keys here are trust and communication.

Another way we learn about doctors is through word of mouth. We ask family, friends, or co-workers for referrals. If overuse injuries are prevalent in your field, ask others who have had similar problems about their experiences, good or bad reactions, successes and failures in treatment, etc.

Some doctors are preceded by their reputations, through their publications, appearances at seminars, or even advertisements. You may hear that a certain doctor is the very best in the state, country, or even world, and he may indeed have a high degree of technical proficiency. But when choosing a physician, technical proficiency may not be enough. Is the doctor also empathetic, compassionate, and patient enough to allow an injured person to follow a less than traditional program? Is he aware and up-to-date about the newest and most innovative methods of treatment? Do you feel good about working with this physician, and entrusting your health to him?

If you are injured on the job, you may be required to see your employer's designated physician. Workers' Compensation carriers and other insurance companies may require you to undergo examinations by their own doctors (see Chapter Eight for more information on this subject). You may want to consider the objectivity of health practitioners who are employed by industries or insurance companies. Is a large percentage of the physician's practice derived from those companies? It is doubtful that a physician would jeopardize a patient's health unnecessarily however, there may be a slant to her philosophy, particularly when the injury is work-related. My personal experience with physicians hired by insurance companies to evaluate my condition have ranged from pleasant to nightmarish, and although I still believe that each physician should be given the benefit of the doubt in terms of his or her objectivity and ability to put the patient's welfare first, the two or three I've met that came with an obvious bias have taught me that as patients we need to be aware of where our caregivers' loyalties lie.

We want doctors and health care professionals who are open-minded, informed, skilled at what they do, and always keeping our best interests at heart. And last, but not least, we want to feel good about our doctors. And that, once the physician's expertise and competence have been established, should be your main criterion when selecting a health care practitioner. You should feel comfortable enough with your doctor to ask questions and have them answered simply and politely, without feeling patronized or rushed. After all, in a sense the doctor is the employee of the patient. You are paying for a service—the doctor is working for *you*.

The Initial Consultation

When you have selected a health care practitioner for an initial consultation, call the office for an appointment. If you are experiencing pain or discomfort, be sure to let the receptionist know when you call. When you arrive for your appointment, expect to spend some time filling out paperwork—the last thing a Carpal Tunnel Syndrome sufferer needs! Ask that the paperwork be sent to you prior to the initial appointment so you can type it or at least fill it out at your own pace. You will be asked if the injury is work-related, and how you plan to pay for the visit. Some health care professionals offer an initial consultation at no charge. If you don't ask, you'll never know.

At the office, you will be called in to see the doctor or therapist, at which point you should be asked about your health history and current complaint(s), and given a thorough physical examination. Refer to Chapter Three for a list of the most common diagnostic tests, and if they are not performed, ask why. I was once sent for a disability evaluation by a physician hired by Social Security, to determine my eligibility for benefits. They took an x-ray and did an *eye* exam. In two weeks I received notice that my claim was denied based on this doctor's examination. He never once touched my hands.

Be prepared to give complete and concise answers to the doctor's questions about your condition. Are your fingers tingling, or is it more like a reduction in their sensitivity? Is the pain in your wrist constant? Intermittent? Sharp? Throbbing? Burning? Are your symptoms worse after activity? At night? Does ice relieve the pain? Heat? Rest? This information is important in assisting your physician in making an accurate diagnosis, so be sure to do your part by providing her with a complete description of how you are feeling. Use the checklist in Appendix A to thoroughly document how you are feeling.

When your examination is complete, you should have the chance to ask some questions of your own. Some examples:

- What is your experience in treating repetitive strain injuries?
- What kinds of cases have you treated and what were the results?
- Do you refer many of your patients out for surgery? Physical therapy?
- What is your criteria for change or stoppage of treatment?
- What do you consider to be the results of successful treatment?

Don't be afraid to ask questions—your doctor should not become defensive or angry when asked to explain his or her criteria (and if they do, you may want to look elsewhere for your health care). The doctor should be willing to discuss these questions and listen to your considerations as well. And don't be alarmed if your physician is initially unsure of your diagnosis. Repetitive strain injuries commonly take some time and investigation in order to come up with an accurate and complete diagnosis. Your doctor may first need to review the results of your EMG, x-rays, or other lab tests, as well as your previous medical records.

Some other things to consider when choosing a health care professional:

- Is the doctor concerned with uncovering the cause of the injury to help you prevent it from recurring?
- Is a program of *rehabilitation* part of the treatment?
- Be very careful if *conservative* care is ruled out right away. Cortisone shots and surgery are not the miracle cures they are sometimes purported to be. There are some severe cases of CTS when immediate surgery is an appropriate recommendation; however, these cases are uncommon and in most instances some form of conservative care is the initial treatment of choice.

We need straight answers to help us make appropriate decisions in health care. In a perfect world, we could visit a doctor who would, after a thorough examination, say, "Ms. Smith, you have evidence of nerve compression in your wrist. Here is what I am trained to do to relieve it. If, however, after a determined length of time I am unable to help you, I will assist you in any way I can in finding other options in treatment which may prove more appropriate in your case. Ask me any questions you like, and I will do my best to give you a complete and objective answer." Imagine the pressure that would relieve, from both the doctor *and* the patient. The physician would not have to be God-like, with all the answers. You would feel comfortable putting your trust in her, knowing your welfare comes first. There are health care professionals out there like that. I know—my own doctor is one, and I've met many more in my eleven years of living with and researching Carpal Tunnel Syndrome. These are the kinds of doctors that we all deserve. Open-minded, informed, secure, and with the patient's well-being at heart. Don't settle for less, and don't give up until you find one.

Obtaining a Second Opinion

Obtaining a second opinion may be a good idea, especially if for any reason you don't feel completely comfortable with your doctor or her diagnosis. You may get the name of another doctor in the same type of specialty—if you saw a chiropractor, see another chiropractor. If you talked to an orthopedist, see another orthopedist. For the most objective evaluation, find the new doctor on your own rather than asking for a referral from your first physician. Let both doctors make an objective diagnosis about your condition and recommendations for treatment.

Once you get an opinion from one specialty of health practitioner (M.D., chiropractor, osteopath, acupuncturist, etc.), you can also inquire into a different type of care. Don't be alarmed if you find there are disagreements between the different specialties. A medical doctor may or may not be supportive of the care you receive from an acupuncturist, or vice versa. It can be extremely confusing as a patient to be told in no uncertain terms by one type of physician that absolutely *no* other treatment plan can be effective, but that happens. "Who's right?" is a question I've heard time and time again from frustrated patients. There is no simple answer. There is something of value to be learned from a variety of health care practitioners, in whatever specialty they practice. Most often, patients find the most effective treatment involves a *combination* of techniques—traditional medical care with massage, chiropractic with homeopathy, etc. Look for a primary-care health professional who is open-minded enough to discuss any and all ideas you have about treatment. It is your job to determine what works best for you, and it is important to explore all your options—the treatment you ultimately choose affects your future and quality of life, and is worth the extra trouble.

A One-Month Trial for Mild Symptoms

If EMG testing is negative, it is safe to say there is probably not significant damage to the median nerve yet. A short, one-month trial on a conservative treatment program should not jeopardize the nerve or cause irreversible damage. You and your physician can choose some specific goals, outline a treatment plan, then re-test in one month to see if there are any changes. If your symptoms improve, great! Continue treatment until symptoms are gone, then begin a strengthening and stretching program to rehabilitate the arm, and work on modifying your work environment if necessary to prevent the injury from recurring.

If your symptoms plateau for four to six weeks, discuss ways to address the remaining symptoms with your doctor. If treatment brings no improvement, it may be time to try something less conservative.

Your Responsibilities

Even the best doctor in the world cannot help you if you don't commit one hundred percent to following the recommended treatment program. When I asked health care professionals to tell me some reasons treatment plans failed, one answer came up again and again: "patient non-compliance." The patients just didn't follow the prescribed treatment plan. Stretching, warm-up exercises, icing painful spots, and/or lifestyle changes are *your* responsibility, and your physician can't do those things for you. Often patients go to a doctor expecting to be made well—given a magic pill that will heal them in a day or so. Carpal Tunnel Syndrome and overuse injuries don't develop overnight, nor will they disappear in an instant. Anti-inflammatory medication or a shot of cortisone can bring quick relief, but the injury is virtually guaranteed to progressively worsen if changes in work and personal habits aren't made, or if underlying health concerns are not addressed. It is vital that you see yourself and your physician as a team, both actively working toward the same goal.

CHAPTER FIVE

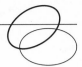

Options in Treatment

"Chiropractic care for Carpal Tunnel Syndrome? What's next . . . coffee enemas and Laetrile?"

"Acupuncture cured my CTS."

"Surgery to relieve CTS is as simple as cutting a belt that's too tight. It works!"

"All you need is B6. It's like a miracle."

Each of these statements was made to me by someone with personal experience with Carpal Tunnel Syndrome, either as a physician or patient. Each was sincere and enthusiastic, eager to share what they believed worked. I heard many more opinions, in wholehearted support or angry condemnation of one treatment or another. In all these years I've yet to hear a story or read a study that can sway me from my own philosophy regarding CTS—no two cases are exactly the same. Different treatments work for different people.

There is no ONE "cure" for Carpal Tunnel Syndrome!

Each of us has a different physiology—different ways of developing symptoms, different ways of healing. There are lots of ideas out there for relieving symptoms of CTS, from surrounding the afflicted limb with quartz crystals to injecting steroids into the wrist. It sometimes takes time and a little detective work to find what will work for you. This chapter looks at some of the common therapies you'll probably come across in your search for effective therapy for relieving your Carpal Tunnel Syndrome.

Medical Doctors

Most of us are familiar with the practice of traditional Western medicine—the diagnosis and treatment of disease and maintenance of health by a licensed medical doctor, often using medication and/or surgery. The first doctor you see about your symptoms may be your family doctor or perhaps the physician to whom you are referred by your employer. These doctors may or may not be familiar with overuse injuries. Another option is to make an appointment with an M.D. who *specializes* in hand/wrist disorders, repetitive strain injuries, or musculoskeletal disorders. The following medical specialists may be able to help you:

• *Physiatrists:* Licensed M.D.s specializing in physical medicine and rehabilitation, physiatrists treat a wide variety of acute and chronic musculoskeletal disorders. They do not perform surgery, and may be able to offer a more diverse array of therapies designed to assist patients in returning to their individual level of maximum functioning. Physiatrists often have access to the most sophisticated and effective diagnostic and therapeutic equipment, and while they do focus on symptom relief, prevention and rehabilitation and strengthening are important parts of treatment as well.

• *Neurologists:* These are medical doctors trained in the diagnosis and treatment of disorders of the nervous system. Carpal Tunnel Syndrome involves the nerves of the upper extremities, and neurologists are generally well-equipped to accurately diagnose disorders of this type.

• *Orthopedists/Orthopedic Surgeons:* These physicians deal with many conditions of the bones, muscles, ligaments, and tendons, including Carpal Tunnel Syndrome. In cases where an injury does not respond to conservative care for a reasonable length of time, the patient may then be referred to a physician in this specialty to determine whether surgical intervention may be needed.

- *Rheumatologists:* These doctors are specialists in disorders of the joints, muscles and associated structures, such as arthritis, degenerative joint disease, and myositis (inflammation of muscle tissue).

Medical doctors who work in the area of sports medicine sometimes also have experience in treating CTS and work closely with physical therapists in rehabilitating the injured limb, as do M.D.s who specialize in pain management or occupational medicine. A comprehensive treatment plan will not only help repair the injury but also help to strengthen the arms and the entire upper body to prevent the condition from recurring. Choosing a doctor who shares your goal of regaining function and mobility, not simply relieving symptoms quickly, is your best bet.

Medication

Medications, such as aspirin, ibuprofen, and the newer naproxen sodium may be recommended by your medical doctor to ease pain and numbness. The class of drugs known as NSAIDs (non-steroidal anti-inflammatory drugs) *can* effectively relieve symptoms. Aspirin, ibuprofen and naproxen inhibit the body's production of *prostaglandins,* a substance that triggers pain. But read the warning labels that accompany these drugs—prolonged use (longer than three to five days) may do more harm than good. Stomach upset, prolonged bleeding time, gastrointestinal bleeding, and impaired kidney function are a few of the known side effects of aspirin and ibuprofen. Prescription muscle relaxants or narcotic pain relievers can cause dizziness and nausea, and some are dangerously addictive. Be sure to ask your physician about any medication he recommends. Read the package insert on any medication you plan to use. Ask about drug interactions if you are using more than one medication. Even if symptoms subside considerably, it is still important for you to make changes in the habits that caused the injury in the first place. Medication can be helpful in relieving symptoms of pain and tingling while you pursue physical therapy or restructuring your workstation, but prolonged use can be dangerous. In other words, medication can help get you over the hump until you are able to bring the symptoms under control.

One warning to take into consideration: beware of feeling so much "better" that you jump right out and spend six hours straight at the keyboard. The symptoms have been masked, but the problem has not been eliminated. Medication should not be seen as a "cure" for an injury caused or affected by overuse.

If you are given a medication to take for your symptoms, ask the following questions:

- What will this medication do for my symptoms?
- What are the normal side effects of this medication? What side effects are considered unusual?
- How long should I take this medication?
- Are there any drug interactions I should be aware of? Food restrictions? Should I take it on a full stomach?
- Is there a package insert I can read to learn more?

Be sure that your doctor is aware of any other medication you are using, allergies you may have, or other health concerns. If you can't get your questions answered, leave and find another doctor who will honor your desire to learn about your condition and treatment. Take notes, ask for package inserts, and learn about what you are putting into your body.

I recommend that you purchase one of the many good reference books describing the uses and side effects of prescription and over-the-counter drugs, such as a recent *Physician's Desk Reference*. Most large bookstores have many such books to choose from, in a variety of price ranges. You can probably also find helpful information in your public library, free of charge. Do become informed about any medications you are using, and don't be afraid to ask questions of your doctor or pharmacist. Pharmacists are an often-overlooked but excellent source of help if you are not sure about the effects or proper usage of a medication.

More about NSAIDs

Since 1899, aspirin has been one of the best-known pain relievers and anti-inflammatories. However, the large group of medications known as non-steroidal anti-inflammatories includes many other drugs which you may hear about or have prescribed for you by your doctor. NSAIDs include:

diclofenac (Voltaren)

diflunisal (Dolobid)

etodolac (Lodine)

fenoprofen (Nalfon)

ibuprofen (Advil, Motrin, Nuprin)

indomethacin (Indocin)

ketoprofen (Orudis)

meclofenamate (Meclomen)

mefenamic acid (Ponstel)

nabumetone (Relafen)

naproxen (Aleve, Anaprox, Naprosyn)

oxyphenbutazone (Oxalid)

phenylbutazone (Azolid, Butazolidin)

suprofen (Profenol)

tolmetin (Tolectin)

These medications vary in their uses and forms.

What about Acetaminophen?

Marketed under brand names like Datril and Tylenol, acetaminophen is an effective analgesic (pain reliever), but does not reduce inflammation like aspirin, ibuprofen, or the other non-steroidal anti-inflammatories.

Cortisone Injections

Cortisone (a type of *steroid*—a strong anti-inflammatory medication) injections may be recommended by your physician, usually providing temporary relief. Eighty percent of patients will feel an improvement in pain and numbness; however, one year later only twenty percent of those patients will remain pain-free.[4] Like other anti-inflammatory medications, cortisone injections should be viewed as a *temporary* measure to relieve acute symptoms, not as a cure. Long-term usage of cortisone can do more harm than good side effects include elevated blood pressure, menstrual disturbances, and muscle weakness.

---

4. *Annals of Physical Medicine* 6(7):287-294, 1962.

Surgery

If damage to the median nerve has progressed to the point where more conservative methods fail, your physician may suggest surgery as soon as possible to relieve the pressure on the nerve, allowing it to function properly again. There is a legitimate fear that the longer the nerves are irritated, the less the chances for successful surgery and recovery. For patients presenting with longstanding symptoms of numbness, pain, or atrophy (wasting away) of the muscles, available treatment options may very well be limited to surgical intervention.

Patients considering surgery are commonly referred to orthopedic surgeons, neurosurgeons, or even plastic surgeons. Under local or general anesthetic, the transverse ligament is cut and released, relieving the pressure on the median nerve. The incision is typically about two inches long. Recovery time varies, depending on the degree of damage to the median nerve and the technique used by the surgeon. There may be some discomfort following the procedure, but this normally does not last for more than a few days. If you are asleep under general anesthetic during the surgery, you will need some time to recover from its effects as well. You will wake up with a large bandage or cast covering the hand and wrist, which will be removed in a week or two by your doctor and replaced with a lighter gauze bandage. The scar from this type of surgery is barely noticeable in most cases.

A newer technique is performed by inserting a tube beneath the carpal tunnel through a small half-inch incision, winding a viewing arthroscope and cutting tool through the tube to the site of the problem, then cutting away the tissue that is pressing down upon the median nerve. Unlike the traditional open surgical approach, which requires the surgeon to make a larger incision to expose the compressed nerve, the new "closed" procedure causes little scarring and a quicker recovery.

Some of the controversy surrounding the option of surgery as the treatment of choice for relieving the symptoms of Carpal Tunnel Syndrome is related to timing. Is surgery best saved as a last resort, after conservative treatments have been tried and found ineffective, or is it best to perform the surgical release as soon as possible after diagnosis? There are pros and cons to both arguments, and plenty of doctors and patients on both sides of the fence. On one hand, the idea of quick resolution, prevention of further deterioration, and the relatively simple nature of the surgery itself appeals to some, while for others the risks of surgery and the idea of potential failure (or in a few cases, a worsening of the condition) lead them to try other means to relieve the symptoms. Once again, there can be no singular clear-cut answer for every case.

An article published in 1991 in *The Journal of the American Medical Association* raises alarming questions about surgical intervention for Carpal Tunnel Syndrome. A full *fifty-seven percent* of post-surgical patients in their study reported a recurrence of their symptoms, such as numbness and pain. 1994 study by Washington University in St. Louis, Missouri found that in fact, surgery for relief from the symptoms of Carpal Tunnel Syndrome is *not* often necessary or recommended. Their theory, recently published in *The Journal of Hand Surgery,* asserts that unnatural posture, tight muscles in the neck, shoulders and upper back, lack of exercise, and poor physical condition also contribute to the occurrence of symptoms like pain and numbness, and these problems are not addressed by performing surgery on the wrist. The study involved teaching patients to restore balance to the muscles through stretching and strengthening, and most patients reported long-term relief. While not a cure for everyone suffering from CTS symptoms (surgery is still considered necessary in some specific cases), this study certainly supports what many "holistic" health care professionals have been saying all along—it is vital to look at the *whole person,* including posture, work habits, and overall fitness level, when determining both cause and treatment for each individual case of CTS.

If your doctor recommends surgery, discuss your options. Is immediate surgery necessary, or could a more conservative course of treatment be attempted first without risk of further damage to the nerve? Ask questions perhaps even seek a second opinion before making a final decision. As with *any* medical procedure, a successful result cannot be guaranteed. Surgery to release the transverse ligament can fail for a variety of reasons. In his booklet on CTS, Dr. Ray Wunderlich, Jr., an M.D. in St. Petersburg, Florida (see below), discusses a few of the possible causes for failure of the surgical method of treatment to relieve the symptoms of Carpal Tunnel Syndrome, including scarring, incomplete transection of both bands of the carpal tunnel ligament, and progression of the inflammation that impinges on the median nerve. Interestingly, Dr. Wunderlich found that most often the patient was actually suffering from what he calls "pseudo-CTS"—patients with hand symptoms arising from hypertonic muscles, nerve entrapment and trigger points in the *arm, shoulder, and neck.* Again, the need for an accurate and complete diagnosis is demonstrated.

Talk to your doctor about your particular case. He will be able to examine the results from your diagnostic tests and give you some idea of your chances for a successful recovery.

"My surgery went very well and I noticed a huge improvement right away. After a month off to recover, though, I went back to work and within a year had developed CTS again. I didn't really get well until I modified my work habits, posture and diet."

"When I woke up from the surgery, I immediately noticed that the feeling in my fingers had returned. Recovery was easy—I'd been in so much pain before the operation I barely felt discomfort from the stitches and the incision."

"Even though I had bilateral surgeries, I still have tingling fingertips at times but no 'asleep hands.' When I adjust my posture, the tingling goes away soon after."

Talking With Ray Wunderlich, Jr., M.D.

In early 1994 I began a correspondence with Dr. Ray Wunderlich (see above), and I found his booklet on the natural treatment of CTS to be well-researched and informative. It contains plenty of scientific theory coupled with an open-minded investigation of alternative causes and treatment of CTS and similar conditions. Dr. Wunderlich was kind enough to answer a few questions for me.

TC: Dr. Wunderlich, what inspired you to write your book?

RW: I saw so many patients that were being operated on who were not getting the long-term results that they wanted. We needed to develop the supportive nutritional and alternative measures as *first-line* approaches, reserving surgery for a later option.

TC: What types of health care professionals may specialize in treatment of CTS?

RW: Categories that may be called upon for investigation could be medical physicians (orthopedists, general physicians, internists, neurologists, etc.), physical therapists, massage and neuromuscular therapists, chiropractic and osteopathic physicians, acupuncturists, radiologists, nutritionists, reflexologists, and perhaps others.

TC: What diagnostic tests do you recommend to obtain an accurate and complete diagnosis?

RW: Nerve conduction studies and magnetic resonance imaging (MRI) of the wrist are often desirable.

TC: Do you ask your patients to make any changes in their activities, lifestyle, or diet?

RW: All patients are asked to improve their diet and lifestyle as background factors. Supplements are usually needed.

TC: At what stage of Carpal Tunnel Syndrome should a patient consider surgery?

RW: In uncomplicated cases of CTS of recent onset, I urge initial, conservative, natural therapies. I reserve surgery for those patients who fail to respond to those measures. If symptoms worsen, I would quickly invoke the services of a surgeon. It is foolish to blindly persist in natural therapies that fail to improve the condition. Delay in relieving the pressure on the median nerve can lead to lasting loss of function. The late stages often require surgery, while early stages do not. However, some patients may need surgery even in the middle stages.

TC: Any suggestions for people in "high-risk" occupations?

RW: Be sure to do forearm, arm, hand, and finger exercises. Have regular body massages, deep muscular or neuromuscular therapy massages, at least once a month. Also, *regular* chiropractic care is a must.

Please see Appendix B for more information on Dr. Wunderlich's publications under "Books".

Natural Medicine

Less traditional methods of treatment may not be as familiar, but they have proven successful in treating many cases of CTS. Medications and surgical intervention are not appropriate for every diagnosis of repetitive strain injury.

Whether you call it alternative, holistic, or natural medicine, there are numerous health practitioners who employ techniques other than drug therapy and surgery to help their patients get well. And rather than seeing the choice between standard and alternative medicine as an "either-or" situation, different healing professions *can* work together, complementing each other. The idea of mixing typical Western medicine with the more "holistic" approaches of, say, acupuncture, homeopathy, or chiropractic, is a new one. But it may be the most effective way to successfully serve *all* of a patient's needs in the treatment of injury or disease. There are times when medicine or surgery are not enough, and supplemental care in a more systemic, whole-body mode will turn the case around. Likewise, an acupuncturist may refer a client out for surgery when an injured nerve isn't responding to treatment. Finding a physician or therapist with an open mind and awareness of the ways in which various specialties can enhance, rather than compete with, each other is a powerful first step toward recovery from injury.

Chiropractic

Chiropractic is the largest natural healing profession in the United States (47,000 practitioners in 1992). Chiropractors believe that many musculoskeletal problems can be caused by different types of pressure on the nervous system, and that the loss of normal nerve activity can also lead to disorders of certain organic systems. Carpal Tunnel Syndrome involves the nerves of the wrist, but those nerves connect all the way up through the arm, shoulder, and neck. If there is pressure on a nerve in the spine, the effects can reach all the way down to the fingertips.

A chiropractic physician restores the nervous system to normal by "adjusting" the patient—relieving pressure by manipulating a particular joint that is *fixated,* or "stuck," back in the proper direction, removing the cause of nerve irritation and enabling the nervous system to heal or regulate itself.

According to chiropractor Dr. Michael Madden, there are generally two schools of thought related to chiropractic care. Some chiropractors are the traditionalists, or "straights," limiting their treatment to manipulation of the spine. On the other side are the liberalists, or "mixers," who employ a variety of techniques in addition to manipulation—massage, electrical therapy like ultrasound and interferential current therapy, nutrition, homeopathy.

Subluxations (misalignments of the spine) or fixations in the wrist, elbow, shoulder, or neck can interfere with the nerves in that area. Problems originating above the wrist can affect the nerves going to the wrist. Cervical spine (neck) problems especially are often noted with Carpal Tunnel Syndrome.

Adjusting the vertebrae in the spine relieves the primary compression, then the arm and wrist can be treated to improve function and reduce

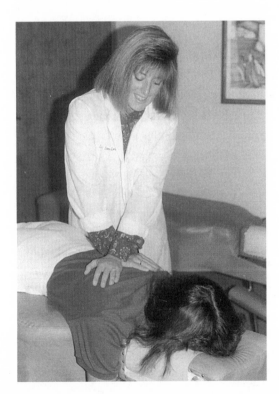

Figure 15. Chiropractor
Dena Lendrum at work

symptoms. Medical research has shown that the chance of a successful outcome from CTS surgery is greatly reduced if there is also a problem in the neck that is left untreated, so chiropractic physicians believe it is vital to look beyond the wrist when treating CTS.

Some Doctors of Chiropractic use their hands to perform an adjustment, while others use instruments. Most rely on orthodox methods of diagnosis, such as the use of x-rays and orthopedic and neurological tests, and may employ physical therapy, including massage and ultrasound, when indicated. A visit to the chiropractor is pleasant for most patients. And though the "cracking" sound you may hear while being adjusted can be unnerving at first, there is often a feeling of relief and "loosening up" afterward. If not, tell your doctor. Medicare, Workers' Compensation, and many private insurance companies will cover the cost of chiropractic treatment. Your chiropractor may also work with you on diet, exercise, and lifestyle, with the idea that overall health greatly affects the process of recovery from injury.

Talking with Dr. Paul Kratka

During the course of my research on repetitive strain injuries I've had the privilege of coming to know a few health care professionals who stood above the rest in terms of their dedication to helping patients recover from repetitive strain injuries. Dr. Paul Kratka is one such individual, and the many patients who have regained the use of their hands through his care will agree. I heard from many of them personally. Dr. Kratka took time out from his busy chiropractic practice in Carlsbad, California, to answer some of my questions in an extensive interview that offers a wealth of information for anyone experiencing the symptoms of CTS.

TC: Dr. Kratka, you're widely known as the "Carpal Tunnel Doctor." How did your interest in helping people with CTS come about?

PK: While in chiropractic school I was trained in a particular chiropractic technique called Gonstead. It differs significantly from other chiropractic methods in that it is very meticulous and specific in the examination and analysis of a patient's problem and the method in which the patient is adjusted. It also includes comprehensive training in the examination, evaluation and adjusting of the extremities, which include the shoulder, elbow, wrist, knee, TMJ [temporomandibular joint], etc. Because of my training in extremities, as my practice grew I began to see more patients with wrist and hand problems. I found patients with CTS were experiencing lasting correction by adjusting the wrist in addition to the spine to relieve the nerve irritation. I soon realized that patients suffering from Carpal Tunnel Syndrome were in great need of *corrective* care instead of the medically-oriented palliative care.

TC: In your booklet "Carpal Tunnel Syndrome: Correcting the Cause," you talk about the "double crush phenomenon." Can you elaborate?

PK: I think this is one of the most important concepts for people to understand. Carpal Tunnel Syndrome is a collection of symptoms which can include pain, numbness, tingling, and weakness of the hand and wrist. CTS is by definition a nerve entrapment where the nerves to the hand are being "entrapped" along their pathway to the hand. The term "double crush" means that there are two areas of nerve entrapment occurring along the course of the nerve, one "upstream" and one "downstream". What actually causes the symptoms are these two areas of nerve irritation, one occurring at the neck where the nerves to the hand originate and another occurring further downstream at the wrist. It is the additive effect of these two nerve irritations that creates Carpal Tunnel Syndrome. The existence of cervical neuritis [irritation] is widely referenced in the medical literature as a consistent finding in CTS patients, and in fact it is difficult to find an article about CTS which *doesn't* discuss double crush. Yet medically it is rarely addressed or treated. It is my personal opinion based upon my clinical observations that sixty to seventy percent of the symptoms associated with CTS are caused by cervical nerve irritation and that only thrity to forty percent are caused by nerve irritation at the wrist. This is evidenced by the many people with CTS who experience successful results under the care of a chiropractor who only adjusts their spine and never their wrists.

TC: What can the patient expect in a visit to a chiropractor?

PK: That is the most difficult question to address because each patient is so different. Some patients have had their problem for one month, others for years; some only have tingling in one hand, others have pain and weakness in both hands; some have had a series of cortisone injections or perhaps one or more wrist surgeries; occupations, hobbies, and past injury/medical histories very greatly. All of these factors influence the outcome of any type of care including chiropractic care. Our current health care system is based upon quick symptom relief, usually utilizing drugs. Therefore, patient expectations have developed along those lines. Unfortunately, most health problems do not lend themselves to "quick fixes." Most patients also want definite time frames and expect their symptoms to improve in a systematic fashion. Unfortunately, the human body is not mechanistic and therefore doesn't lend itself to such predictions or prognosis. The human body is extremely vitalistic and varies tremendously from individual to individual and from day to day. Perhaps one of the most frustrating things for some patients is that they will often experience exacerbations [worsening] during the course of their care. They have been conditioned to expect continuous improvement and when it doesn't happen as they expect, they become discouraged.

I always explain to each patient that there are three phases of chiropractic care: First is relief care; the goal is to reduce and eliminate a patient's symptoms. The first phase of care usually takes from one to sixteen weeks, and the patient is adjusted three to four times per week.

The second phase is stabilization care during this phase the patient's symptoms are minimal or gone altogether and yet their care continues to stabilize their condition so it won't recur. Stabilization takes from two to ten months, and the patient is adjusted one to two times per week.

Finally, there is wellness or preventative care: this is when the patient is asymptomatic and has remained so for some time and wishes to take a preventative approach to their health care. There is no time frame and the patient is usually checked every two to six weeks.

It is important for patients to understand that it was a process (i.e., time) that created their condition and it will be a process (i.e., time) that corrects it. And that they will probably experience some ups and downs along the way. Persistence and perseverance are often the determining factors in a patient's success.

Finally, there is the limitation of time and matter. For example, if a patient has severe degenerative changes present in their spine, had previous surgeries which resulted in significant scar tissue, or damaged structures and tissues (i.e., nerves, tendons, etc.), chiropractic care may not achieve the results they are looking for. That's not to say that patients who have had surgeries or have advanced degeneration in their spine won't benefit from chiropractic care many do every day. It's important to put things in perspective. Chiropractic works in all diseases and conditions; however, it does not work in all cases of all diseases and conditions.

TC: What changes do you ask your patients to make in their activities, lifestyle, diet, etc.?

PK: During the initial relief care phase I will often recommend to the patient that they refrain from any activities which may inhibit the corrective process. This may include avoiding such things as needlepoint, bartending, gardening, etc.. However, at some point we (the patient and I) need to find out if what we're doing is going to be successful under the conditions which created their problem. Usually during the stabilization phase, I will suggest that the patient gradually begin to perform the activities that led to their problem or aggravated it in the past. It allows the patient and I to determine what level of correction has been accomplished up to that point. This is often very subjective but it begins the process of defining parameters with which patients can get on with their lives.

There are also some recommendations that can be applied to all qualified patients. A partial list of these include the following:

- If the patient spends much of their day on the telephone, utilizing a head-set, is important to avoid creating chronic neck problems and to achieve stability to their correction.
- If the patient spends any significant portion of their day using a computer, it is important they set up their workstation ergonomically so that the monitor is directly in front of them and at eye level; that the keyboard is at a proper (neutral) height for their wrist/hand positioning, and that there is a *wide* wrist support extended off the keyboard. If they use a mouse, instead change to using a trackball (i.e., Logitech) which is also positioned at a neutral wrist/hand position.
- Wear wrist splints at night if their symptoms wake them at night or are aggravated by sleeping.

- Wear wrist supports (different from wrist splints) during the day while working or performing their daily activities during the relief care and stabilization care phases.
- Avoid sleeping on the stomach; sleep only on the back or the side, using a cervical pillow. I recommend using cervical pillows made of polyester fiber fill, not foam; including the following brands: Linear Gravity pillow (Anabolic Labs), Tri-Core, D-Core.
- Take a high-quality vitamin B6 supplement (Standard Process, Metagenics); vitamin B6 has been shown to facilitate the healing of injured nerves.
- If the patient engages in an activity or occupation in which they are standing or working in a stressful position for prolonged periods (i.e., hairdresser, dental hygienist, etc.), implement a stretching regimen into their daily work and exercise routines (yoga is superior to all types of stretching).

TC: What should a patient look for in selecting a health care practitioner?

PK: If a patient goes to a chiropractor, the chiropractor wants to adjust that patient because that's what a chiropractor does. If a patient goes to an orthopedic or neurosurgeon, they will want to operate because that's what surgeons do. So clearly there is subjective bias built into this situation. That being said, my first recommendation to any patient is to pursue all conservative, non-invasive, non-drug-oriented methods of care *first*. After all, drug therapy (cortisone injections, ibuprofen, naprosyn, etc.) and surgery are options that will always be available and they are not time dependent. (It always surprises me to hear that some people consider drugs or surgery to be conservative and chiropractic or acupuncture to be radical.) Next, I would recommend that the practitioner be someone who specializes in Carpal Tunnel Syndrome, not just a doctor who has bought the latest CTS therapy device. I think physical therapy attempts to relieve symptoms without correcting the cause. The doctor should be a chiropractor who is superior in their clinical competence and who has had extensive training and experience in adjusting extremities and treating CTS patients.

So, how does a patient determine if a doctor they're considering meets these criteria? Call the doctor and ask them. I know this sounds overly simplistic but it works. But, don't call up a doctor and ask, "Do you treat Carpal Tunnel Syndrome?" because they'll probably just say yes. Ask them, "What do you specialize in your practice? What techniques do you use?," etc. If it sounds like the doctor is trying to be everything to everybody, then it probably isn't the right office. If someone calls my office and asks me what I do, I respond that I was trained in the Gonstead method, I take care of babies to seniors, and that I have a Carpal Tunnel Syndrome subspecialty within my practice. If the person is looking for ultrasound, homeopathy, applied kinesiology or something I don't do, rather than coerce them into my office under false pretenses, I refer them to another doctor.

TC: Do you have any advice for people at risk for development of repetitive strain injuries?

PK: First, remember that you are responsible for your health. Your doctor is not responsible for your health, your insurance company is not responsible for your health, *you* are responsible for your health. Your employer is only responsible for preventing and treating work-related injuries. So what does all this mean? It means that you must take control of your health and your situation. If you are presently experiencing any symptoms or if you work in an environment that is causing you to develop any symptoms, don't wait to get help, thinking your problem will go away (the six most common words heard in a chiropractic office are "I thought it would go away"). Immediately seek help from the practitioner of your choice. If it is a work-related injury, know your rights as an employee. For example, in California an employee may predesignate their personal physician or chiropractor for their care in the event that they get hurt on the job; also, if your employer directs you to an industrial medical clinic, you can immediately request to be seen by a chiropractor. These are state laws that very few employees are aware of, yet the law stipulates that it is the employer's legal duty to inform the employee of these rights.

If you presently are not experiencing any symptoms but are at risk for development of repetitive stress injuries, I suggest that you make sure that all preventative and ergonomic precautions are being taken to prevent you from getting injured. This is easier said than done when dealing with an employer because they are often reluctant to spend the time and money to implement these precautions. My suggestion to supermarket cashiers, computer operators, electricians, piano players, etc., is that they better be practicing yoga, or receiving preventative chiropractic care, or somehow taking personal responsibility for their own health. Remember, it is your health and no one is going to protect it as well as you yourself can.

Dr. Kratka is the owner and director of La Mar Chiropractic, a practice which emphasizes preventative care, nutritional therapy, and patient education. Dr. Kratka is a California state-appointed Qualified Medical Examiner, and consults with Workers' Compensation insurance companies and industry on Carpal Tunnel Syndrome and injury prevention programs. He can be personally reached at (619) 930-8039.

Physical Therapy

Physical therapists are highly trained health care professionals who assist in rehabilitation and restoration of normal bodily function after illness or injury through the use of therapeutic exercises, hydrotherapy, and the application of various forms of energy—electrotherapy, ultrasound, and interferential current therapy. Generally, a medical doctor or other health care provider will refer a patient to a physical therapist as part of the treatment plan. Most states require a referral from your doctor allowing you to be treated by a physical therapist. A physical therapist can also teach you about proper work habits, posture, and how you can achieve a more healthy lifestyle. Most patients, myself included, find the experience pleasant and helpful.

Let's start by talking about a few of the tools used in physical therapy.

Ultrasound

Ultrasound uses high-frequency sound waves to increase blood flow to an injured area, to warm muscles, and to relieve pain. Ultrasound can also reduce tissue inflammation and edema (swelling). More effective than simple vibration or heat, ultrasound penetrates deep into the muscles and joints. Combined with other therapies (physical therapy, chiropractic), ultrasound can help to relieve symptoms of CTS when administered by a trained professional.

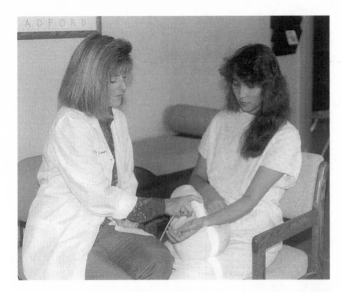

Figure 16. Ultrasound

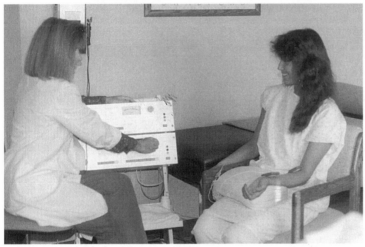

Figure 17. Interferential
current therapy

Interferential Current Therapy

A type of electrical treatment, interferential current therapy has become
quite popular in recent years in the treatment of Carpal Tunnel Syndrome
and other overuse injuries. The medium-frequency current penetrates deep
into the joint or muscle, to increase circulation, reduce swelling and inflammation, stimulate the release of pain-reducing hormones in the body, and
increase overall muscle tone. A session with the interferential unit lasts about

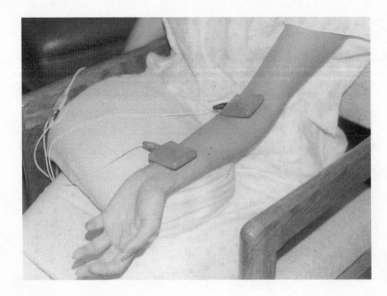

Figure 18. Pads in place for CTS therapy

ten to fifteen minutes in most cases, and the feeling of the electrical pulse is somewhat odd but not uncomfortable. Results can be dramatic, and longer lasting than treatment with ultrasound.

Iontophoresis: More Effective Delivery of Medication?

The RSI Network reports that, according to Iomed Inc. of Salt Lake City, the use of electrical currents to deliver anti-inflammatory medication may be highly effective as a treatment for CTS. Patients participating in a 1992 independent study received three treatments over a period of one week of *iontophoresis,* minute electrical current applied to an electrode which transports drugs through the skin. After the treatment a majority of patients were symptom-free, and three months later sixty-three percent continued to have no or minimal symptoms. Iontophoresis has already been approved by the Food and Drug Administration for treatment of CTS. The company states that iontophoresis eliminates the pain and complications of steroid medication and costs less than surgery. Iomed projects the total cost for treatment to be $200 compared to the $2,500 that would be charged for surgery.

TENS

A small, battery-operated device, wired to electrode patches attached to the patient's skin, the TENS (transcutaneous electrical nerve stimulation) unit is gaining in popularity as an effective pain reliever for all kinds of symptoms. Like acupuncture, the electrical pulses seem to stimulate the body's own natural painkillers. The patient generally feels nothing more than a mild tingling. Ask your doctor or physical therapist if TENS is an option for you.

Talking with Jackie Ross, P.T.

Because physical therapy is so often a part of recovery from repetitive strain injuries (it certainly was for me), I thought it important to include the thoughts of a professional physical therapist—one with extensive experience working with patients suffering from the symptoms of repetitive strain. Jackie Ross has been a physical therapist for 24 years, with a private practice in Manhattan. She acts as a consultant for ergonomic and on-site evaluations.

TC: Jackie, in your work as a physical therapist, what kinds of injuries do you see related to overuse or repetitive trauma?

JR: Some of the injuries I see are Carpal Tunnel Syndrome, Cubital Tunnel Syndrome, tendinitis, tenosynovitis, myositis [muscular inflammation], cervical strains, Thoracic Outlet Syndrome, and fibromyalgia. Of course, some of these diagnoses, i.e., Thoracic Outlet Syndrome and fibromyalgia, seem to be precursors to the problem of hand pain and/or weakness.

TC: What kinds of practitioners make referrals to you, and at what point in the patients' treatment plan?

JR: I receive referrals from internists, occupational medical physicians, orthopedists, physiatrists, osteopathic physicians, chiropractors, and massage therapists. I fortunately have seen the majority of my patients pre-surgically, and only one patient has necessitated surgery post-treatment. I have only seen two patients post-surgically; one for a carpal tunnel release and one for a cubital tunnel release. Only the cubital tunnel release was successful.

TC: What can a patient expect coming in for a session of physical therapy?

JR: When a patient first presents to my office I take a thorough history followed by an evaluation. The evaluation consists of a postural evaluation in the sitting and standing positions, a range of motion test, a strength evaluation, neurological and circulatory evaluations, and an evaluation of the patient in his work environment. Either I do an on-site visit or I have the patient bring in photos of themselves working at their workstations. Most recently, we have been utilizing an on-premise computer workstation. While he or she works at the station, I film the patient on video and monitor their typing techniques. Once the evaluation is complete, therapy begins.

TC: What kinds of therapy do you use in your practice, and what is the patient's role in treatment?

JR: I emphasize two major areas in the patient's treatment: manual releases and exercise. The manual releases I use include massage, strain counterstrain, and myofascial release. I do use modalities such as ultrasound, electric stimulation, and ice to help reduce any inflammation. I've had good results with cervical traction to help reduce pressure on the cervical spine. Treatment is never passive, and the patient takes an active role in his or her rehabilitation. The importance of taking frequent rest and exercise breaks is emphasized. Besides specific exercises to maintain muscular flexibility and a slowly progressive strengthening program, patients are encouraged to become involved in some kind of general conditioning aerobic program. This is particularly important for patients who have fibromyalgia. The other major consideration in the patient's exercise program is that in stretching the tight muscles you do not want to compromise the joint. Almost all RSI patients suffer from some form of ligament laxity in their upper extremities. Some feel better almost immediately due to simple changes at their workstations, frequent breaks, and simple contract-relax exercises to the larger muscles of the shoulder girdle in the initial stages of therapy.

TC: Can you offer any feedback from your experience on the variety of treatments available for CTS?

JR: I've had patients who received relief from acupuncture and biofeedback. Both of these techniques help to reduce pain, but in and of themselves will not solve the problem unless modifications at work are made and appropriate exercises are done.

TC: What advice can you give to patients in the various stages of CTS?

JR: The best advice I can give to both patients and other health care practitioners is to recognize the problem early on. The sooner the patient begins a course of treatment, the shorter the duration and longer-lasting the results. If a patient feels dissatisfied with the results of any therapy program or medical treatment, they should seek help from other sources.

TC: How can patients optimize their chances for a successful outcome?

JR: The patient should become actively involved in all aspects of his/her treatment. They should be able to openly discuss the course of treatment, the prognosis, etc., with their provider of care.

TC: What can a person at risk for development of a repetitive strain injury do to prevent injury?

JR: There are some people who are more susceptible to this type of injury. Hypermobility and forward head posturing are two distinct characteristics which almost all RSI patients exhibit. Recognizing this, a computer user may have to from the onset become aware of the proper ergonomics and be placed on a preventative exercise program to guarantee proper usage of larger muscle groups.

Osteopathy

The system of health care known as osteopathy was founded in the late 1800's by Dr. Andrew Taylor Still. Osteopaths support the theory, as do chiropractors, that achieving a structural balance will bring about healing. Osteopathic physicians (D.O.s) undergo a traditional medical education, which is then followed by additional coursework emphasizing the muscular and skeletal systems. Like chiropractors, osteopaths use manipulation of the spine to correct injuries or imbalances within the neuro-muscular-skeletal system, but they are also licensed to prescribe medication or perform surgery if needed. In that respect, osteopathic physicians are in the unique position of being able to help the body to heal itself through the use of hands-on manipulative therapy, along with the ability to offer treatment with drugs or surgery if necessary. Osteopaths may also emphasize the importance of exercises and stretches to increase range of motion, thus restoring the full functioning of the blood and lymphatic systems. Osteopathy may not be as well known as other systems of health care, but its unique combination of whole-body care with some of the more traditional allopathic tools make it worth looking into for many patients.

The Healing Power of . . . Magnets?

Imagine a new device that could reduce pain and inflammation, stimulate blood flow, and speed the healing process, all without side effects and at a low cost. Those are some of the claims being made about the use of magnets in cases of acute and chronic pain, such as repetitive stress injuries. Biomagnetics refers to the effects of magnetism on living cells. It is thought that placing biomagnets over injured tissue stimulates blood flow to the area, which in turn speeds healing, reduces muscle spasms, and flushes out waste products. Biomagnets are widely accepted for clinical use in Japan, where they are approved by the Japanese Ministry of Welfare (the equivalent of our FDA). Their acceptance here in the U.S. is not as widespread, although currently both Johns Hopkins Medical School and the Massachusetts Institute of Technology are conducting studies of biomagnetic devices and their effect on injuries.

Acupuncture

One of oldest known systems of medicine in the world, acupuncture has been practiced for at least five thousand years. Acupuncture involves the insertion of very fine needles into specific points on the body. It is believed that acupuncture restores the balance of *ch'i*—the energy that makes up each being's life force. Ch'i flows throughout the body along pathways called **meridians,** and illness occurs when the pathways become blocked. Practitioners of traditional Chinese medicine seek to release this trapped energy and restore the body to health.

In acupuncture therapy, specific points are stimulated to restore balance to the body. Again, with Carpal Tunnel Syndrome treatment is *not* necessarily confined to the hands, wrists, and arms. Treating the neck, back, and shoulders as well will begin to heal the entire length of the injured nerve. Acupuncturists may also use transcutaneous nerve stimulation (TENS), heat treatments, and herbs, not only to heal the injury and relieve symptoms, but to bring about balance to the entire system. The philosophy of Oriental medicine supports the idea that a healthy, balanced system is less prone to injury and disease.

Acupuncture stimulates the release of **endorphins,** the body's own natural pain reliever, from the brain. Does acupuncture hurt? It depends on who you ask. Most patients feel comfortable throughout the treatment—the needles used are extremely fine and generally insertion is painless. A few people report a feeling of mild discomfort as the needle is put into place, but this is usually very brief and followed almost immediately by a feeling of calm and relaxation as the treatment proceeds. The needles may be gently twisted while in place, or heat or a mild electrical current may be applied.

Acupuncture is used to relieve a wide variety of problems from headaches to premenstrual syndrome—even as an anesthetic during surgery. And although its acceptance in the Western world has been slow, many insurance companies will now cover the cost of acupuncture. Acupuncturists are also interested in treating the total person; you will be carefully examined and have an extensive history taken at your first visit. In addition to treatment with needles, you may be given herbs or homeopathic remedies (see Homeopathy in this chapter). Your pulse may be checked at several points throughout your body, and your skin, nails, and even tongue examined in order for the acupuncturist to get a sense of the state of your general health.

Massage

Massage involves stroking and kneading the body to loosen the muscle tissues, increase movement of joints and removal of toxins, and restore the flow of energy. Massage increases blood flow to the muscles, and can aid in reducing the stiffness and swelling that often accompany injury. A massage therapist familiar with overuse-type injuries can work wonders in relieving pain and numbness. Don't be afraid to shop around until you find a therapist with the right touch. There are many types of massage, some gentle, some deep. Swedish, Shiatsu, Trager, Esalen—you may hear lots of exotic-sounding terms for the various techniques used by massage therapists. The type of massage you receive will depend on the therapist's training, background, and personal philosophy. Most massage therapists are an excellent source of information and guidance on injury prevention and home care. And because they, too, work with their hands and arms quite a bit, they often have first-hand knowledge about repetitive strain injuries.

The massage therapist should be experienced enough to be able to adjust her technique to your particular needs, and explain what she is doing and why. Your feedback during the session should be encouraged and welcome. A sensitive massage therapist knows when he's found a sore spot and can help you relax while he kneads away the tension. Often CTS patients find they enjoy a deep massage to help work out the "knots" in their necks and shoulders; however, a gentle approach feels best if you have lots of inflammation, when deep work can actually do more harm than good. Find the technique that works best for you.

The Feldenkrais Method®

The Feldenkrais Method is a system of gentle exercise and hands-on manipulation that, according to Feldenkrais instructor Michael Krugman, encourages more effective posture, breathing, and coordination. Exercises are designed to allow the brain to "re-connect" with the body, and students report an increase in range of motion without strain. Check Appendix B for information on the Feldenkrais Method.

Homeopathy

Homeopathic medicine was founded in the late 18th century by Dr. Samuel Christian Friedrigh Hahnemann, and is based on one simple principle—"like cures like." The homeopath considers the whole person when presented with a set of symptoms. Generally, a great deal of time is spent during the first visit in obtaining an extensive history. Not only the physical but also the patient's emotional and mental processes are considered when making a diagnosis. A remedy is chosen which closely fits all aspects of your symptoms and will stimulate your body to heal itself. The correct remedy is one which produces reactions similar to those the patient is experiencing, activating and strengthening the patient's own system in response to the remedy.

Homeopathic remedies are made from natural substances (flowers, minerals, roots, oils, for example) which are sequentially diluted. The more a substance is diluted, the higher its potency. In other words, according to homeopaths, a minute dose of the correct substance will activate the patient's own defenses to attack the illness. Homeopaths may also make recommendations about diet, lifestyle, or exercise to help you bring your life into balance. Homeopathy can work well in conjunction with most other therapies, even traditional Western medicine. Homeopathic remedies may be taken orally in the form of pills or liquid, or applied topically in ointments and creams. An excellent homeopathic cream for topical application to injured arms and hands is called ***Traumeel*** (check your local natural food store or see Appendix C under Biological Homeopathic Industries, Inc. for ordering information). Homeopathy can provide a gentle way to fine-tune your system into optimal health.

There are many choices in health care available for people with Carpal Tunnel Syndrome and other repetitive strain injuries. It's just a matter of finding the particular method and practitioner that work best for you.

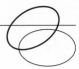

CHAPTER SIX

Stress Management

Your attitude and emotions play a large part in the state of your health. Everyone experiences stress, but why do some people seem to be able to sail through life while others of us become burned out, fatigued, and even succumb to illness as a result of stress?

There is no question that a person living with chronic pain may go through stages of fear, depression, and anger. They may be told the symptoms are "all in their head" or "psychosomatic." Impairment of the use of the hands is devastating, and people suffering from Carpal Tunnel Syndrome often report feelings of helplessness and isolation. They *look* fine, yet they are living with a very real disability. Until recently very little information was available about CTS, and it is still not uncommon for employees to experience a lack of support from supervisors when CTS affects the job performance.

Just as you have learned that physical wellness can only be achieved when you make the time to meet your body's needs, maintaining emotional health requires the same attention. And, like the stretching exercises and self-help techniques you have learned to relieve your physical symptoms, there is a myriad of ways to alleviate tension—yoga, biofeedback, meditation, bodywork such as massage, sports or other physical activities, or just spending time with friends and family can all function as outlets for stress.

Try the techniques discussed in this chapter. When you find one that works for you, set aside a special time every day to practice in a quiet place. Even if you can only spare ten minutes out of your hectic schedule, it is important to schedule a time devoted entirely to taking care of yourself. The best time is early in the morning when you are rested—set the alarm clock fifteen minutes ahead if necessary. Before bed is another good time to unwind by yourself.

Yoga

If the thought of yoga conjures up swamis and incense, welcome to the nineties! Yoga is finally coming into its own as a highly effective form of exercise for both the body and mind. Its postures can strengthen, invigorate, stretch, and/or relax, and nearly everyone can do it.

Health professionals and scientists are beginning to confirm that the regular practice of yoga has a wide range of beneficial effects on a variety of ailments—from weakened immune systems to heart conditions to Carpal Tunnel Syndrome. All you need is a comfortable spot, a floor or level surface, and loose, non-restrictive clothing; however, it's also possible to take a quick yoga break virtually anywhere you are.

Not all yoga poses require bending yourself into a pretzel shape—many are easy to do whatever your abilities are. For example, the Corpse pose is an excellent way to begin or end a sequence of yoga postures, or simply as a way to relax and release stress in itself. Lie on your back, making sure that you have adequate support to allow yourself to completely relax. Place a pillow under your neck to support your head. You may need additional pillows or folded blankets to support your knees or arms. Your lower back should be flat on the floor. Bend your knees if necessary. Breathe deeply and naturally from your *abdomen*—not your chest. To check your breathing, place your hands over your stomach. If you are breathing abdominally, your stomach will rise and fall with each breath. Abdominal breathing may take practice, but it is necessary for a complete exchange of air and total relaxation. Hold this pose for as long as feels comfortable.

It's wise to start off with some formal instruction in yoga. Even a simple pose done incorrectly can cause injury. A yoga teacher can assist you in modifying the postures to accomodate what your body is able to handle. If you are unable to take a class from a qualified instructor, you can certainly benefit from many of the books and videotapes available. I've recommended a few resources for yoga practice in Appendix B.

Progressive Relaxation Exercise

This exercise in progressive relaxation is designed to help you train yourself to feel the difference between relaxation and tension. By understanding what being completely relaxed feels like, you will more easily notice when your muscles are beginning to tighten up in response to stress or fatigue. People who are in pain tend to unconsciously keep their muscles tense all the time, almost as if they were protecting the injured limb.

Try reading the following exercise into a tape recorder so that you can practice without referring back to the book. Sit or lie comfortably, in loose clothing, and remember to take slow, deep breaths throughout the exercise.

Start by focusing your attention on your toes. Clench your toes as tight as you can, and hold for a count of ten. Slowly release the muscles until they are completely relaxed. As you relax, your muscles feel loose and warm.

Next, flex your feet by pointing your toes up and back. You will feel a tightening in your calf muscles. Hold for a count of ten, then slowly release. Feel the muscles in your calves relax.

Tighten the muscles of your buttocks, thighs, and stomach. Feel your legs lift slightly as you count to ten. Slowly release. Continue taking slow, deep breaths as you relax. As you visualize filling your lungs with clean, pure air, see any tension leaving your body each time you exhale.

Next, tense the muscles of your upper body Clench your fists, arms straight out at your sides. Tighten your arms and chest muscles. Hold as you count to ten, then release. Feel the warmth spread throughout your upper body as you relax.

Next, tighten your neck. Push your head back, and clench your jaw and lips tightly together. Hold for a count to ten, then release slowly. Feel all the tension melt away.

Remember to keep breathing, slowly and deeply.

Last, tense the muscles of your face. Open your mouth as wide as you can, as if you are yawning. Tighten your eyes by squeezing them tightly shut. Frown and wrinkle your nose. Hold the muscles tight for a count of ten. Let the tension go as you gently relax.

Positive Mental Imaging

There is growing evidence that our thoughts have a powerful influence on our health. Certainly it is true that holding a calm, pleasant image in the mind can lower heart rate and blood pressure. A visualization to help heal an injured arm might go like this:

First, find a comfortable place where you can totally relax without interruption. You can put on a tape of soothing music, or tape this exercise and play it back. We will focus this exercise on the right arm, but you can adapt this exercise to any part of the body.

Imagine your right arm feeling warm and heavy. Feel the blood moving through the shoulder, elbow, forearm, wrist, hand, and fingers. Your fingers feel warm and relaxed. Now, starting at your shoulder, imagine a ball of white light glowing its way down your arm. The light moves slowly, stopping at any sore spots to melt away the pain.

See the light moving down your upper arm, elbow, forearm, wrist, hand, and fingers. Hold the glowing white ball in your hand for a moment, then let it go, imagining that it is carrying away all the soreness and tension. Feel your arm become light and weightless.

Biofeedback

Biofeedback involves the use of a special machine that, when its sensors are attached to points on the body, can monitor heart rate, temperature, brain wave activity, and muscle tension. Once you are "hooked up" to the machine, it is easy to follow your body's reactions by looking at a digital readout or listening for audio tones that speed up or slow down. You can then begin to identify thought patterns that affect your heart rate, muscle

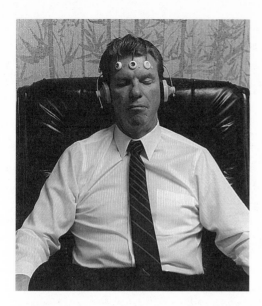

Figure 19. Biofeedback

tension, etc., and train yourself to relax and influence the readings from the machine. Home biofeedback units are available, but formal training is necessary to get a thorough understanding of the techniques involved. Your best bet is a trained professional, at least to get you started on the right foot.

The stretches discussed in Chapter Nine are also helpful in reducing stress, particularly while at work.

Talking with Dr. Linda Haack-Rogers

Dr. Linda Haack-Rogers was a professor of mine when I was working toward my Master's degree in Human Resources Management. She is a licensed clinical psychologist in practice in San Diego, California. In addition to her general practice, Dr. Haack-Rogers has a specialization in sports psychology, and has worked with amateur and professional athletes since 1987.

TC: Dr. Haack-Rogers, what kinds of things do you see happening from a psychological perspective when treating a patient who suffers from a chronic injury?

LHR: A patient with a chronic injury who comes into my office typically has feelings of depression, and within that, feelings of helplessness, hopelessness, failure. Oftentimes, they will feel very overwhelmed by their feelings, and unable to figure out what to do. Sometimes they will have obsessive feelings or thoughts, such as obsessing over their pain—it becomes the focus of their life, so that everything else, family, job or other interests will be restricted to their pain. Sometimes it becomes self-destructive. They start to put themselves down; they start to remove themselves mentally from their daily activities, or their friends or families. The result is a feeling of alienation— "Nobody understands me" or "I'm all alone." Part of that may be true; there may be people who are not suportive, but, part of it may be self-induced. And that's something I [as a psychologist] intend to look at.

TC: When you are working with a patient with this type of injury, what is your relationship with the patient's medical doctor? Does the treating physician refer the patient to you?

LHR: Every situation is different. The patient may have been referred to me by a friend, or by the physician or physical therapist. If the physician has done the direct referral, I tend to have closer communication at that time, because I will contact the referring physician immediately. I think it is important to have the counselor be connected at some point with the physician; first, to establish an understanding of the physican problem. Sometimes the client may distort things in a positive or negative way—they may minimize or maximize their problem, and I go to the physician to really understand the problem clearly. Second, it's important to keep close communication to maximize continuity of care, so you're both on the right track. It wouldn't be good for me to be saying, "It's all in your head," while the doctor is saying "It's all in your hands," or vice versa. It wouldn't be appropriate for the patient to come up with goals that I'm supporting that they are not capable of doing, that would be destructive physically for them. The same is true if they are doing less than they really could do, and holding back rather than continuing to challenge themselves, *if* they're physically capable of doing that and it's needed for the healing process and recovery. Many times athletes who are injured tend to operate more out of fear; their fear will restrain them from truly working back through an injury, and it's important to know the realities of that. The only way you're going to know that is by contacting the physician, and having good communication. It's important to have a least a couple of contacts in the beginning to establish the true background of the problem, then maybe halfway through the treatment to see how things are going, and to see the physician's perspective on the patient's recovery. When I work with athletes, I contact their coaches to get their perspective on the patient's progress. Then of course again at the end of treatment, to see if we've come to a place of healing or achievment of goals, and then I also follow up later. A team approach helps for a speedier recovery.

TC: When you are working with a patient experiencing a long-term, chronic type of injury, what kinds of coping skills might you help a patient learn to assist them in living with the condition and its limitations?

LHR: Thought stopping is a good exercise, particularly with a person who has been obsessing over their pain or feeling negative thoughts toward themselves, feelings of failure. Having the person literally say "Stop," and then rephrase or project into a positive statement. In other words, redirecting their thoughts can be very, very important in any feeling process. We can easily become very negative and it's a spiral that goes down, down, down. Very self-destructive. Thought stopping is a great technique to refocus. For some patients, I have them say it out loud—*"Stop"!* And then you want to replace it with a positive thought.

Another technique to go along with that is goal development. You want to develop some kind of vision or direction for yourself. Without visions or direction, we don't know where to go, how far we've come, when we are a success, nor do we feel good about ourselves. Goal development is really important to help us move out, into a direction we want to get to, and then know your successes along the way. Christopher Reeve is a person who lost everything for the most part in his life, *except* his life, but it's very important in his process back, to develop goals, even if it's a goal of lifting up his pinky, even something as little as that. Some person might say, "Oh, that's not a goal...that's not worth anything." It *is* worth something—you have to measure [success] in terms of what you can achieve, whether big or small compared to somebody else. It's compared to *yourself.* And you have to stay focused on *your* goal development which is specific for you and for your injury. It cannot be compared to somebody else. It takes breaking it down into small sections, into the process of little steps that take you to the larger goal. In goal development you want to have a large goal, and then you can work forward towards that. Sometimes it's better to work backwards and break it down, for example, if the goal is to be able to work a full day again, then you must be able to first work half a day, and then a couple of hours, and then ten minutes—you break it down backwards in very small and specific steps. Write them down, check them off, feel good about it when you've accomplished your goals. Rewrite your goals; do them daily, do them weekly, do them monthly. You'll want to periodically revise your goals.

Another coping skill is the open expression of your feelings. I think it's extremely important to continue to express yourself to people, whether it be your counselor, or ideally, your family and friends. They will then really understand where you are coming from and know you, and you get to express yourself and not hold onto hurt, anger, and resentment, which increases depression. So the better your communication is, one, the stronger your support system will eventually be, because they are going to really understand you and know what you're going through, and two, the more you can focus on where you want to go, and not have all your baggage hold you up.

Another coping skill is meditation. With pain comes tension—a secondary tension where other muscles which are not involved in the injury become tense, sore, and even damaged. We can only hold a fist tight for so long before we eventually fall to exhaustion. That can wear a person out completely, full-body. Even if you are dealing with something which started out as Carpal Tunnel, then eventually the patient could reach the point of saying, "All I want to do is sleep." The whole body has reacted to the initial pain. So, meditation and breathing are very good skills to develop and constantly work on. Meditation isn't something that comes overnight; I recommend that people actually go and get trained. Take a yoga, meditation, or relaxation class. It's basically all the same thing. I'm calling it meditation, but you can also call it visualization or progressive relaxation. Working on meditation will help keep the muscles that you need energized, energized and relaxed, and utilized appropriately. When I work with athletes, it's important that they use the exact muscles that they need to get through their performance, and *not* use their relaxed muscles, which would take from their energy. In working through pain, meditation helps people become more aware of their tense places and their relaxed places. It also helps in visualizing and positive thoughts versus the obsessive or negative thinking. Breathing is the absolute key step in meditation and relaxation. People do forget to breathe. We can easily breathe through pain. In the birthing process, the whole Lamaze technique is based on breathing through pain. Yes, it's still painful to go through childbirth, but you can work *with* your body, rather than against it. If you really work on progressive relaxation or meditation, you can bring yourself from a tense state to a very relaxed one with three deep breaths, if you really work at it. It is something you actually have to practice, and without daily practice you won't be good at it, like anything else.

TC: It sounds like something we can easily do at work, as well.

LHR: Anywhere. Absolutely anywhere, anytime. You're not going to bring attention to yourself. No one's going to say, "What is she doing? How weird!" Everybody breathes.

TC: What about our attitudes as patients—how does attitude affect recovery?

LHR: People can look to physicians for that "quick fix"—for the pill that makes them feel better, for the surgery that will "make it all go away," and I think it's important that you do take personal responsibility for your own healing and your own treatment. Doctors aren't God. I know that they are wonderful, and they have wonderful things to treat conditions that we would have died from years ago, and they do save lives. But they are not omnipotent, in that they don't have answers to everything. Actually, *you* do, because it's your body, and every body is different. To rely on pills or surgery isn't the truth about healing. Healing comes from within. When you rely on something artificial outside of your body, you tend to have higher consequences, such as side effects from medications, addictions, things like that. Then you feel a sense of greater loss and helplessness. When you do work on things that are more of an internal nature, you actually have deeper healing that goes on. We know that we can build up our immune systems through psychological means; meditation, visualizations. We have people experiencing spontaneous recoveries that doctors don't have the answer for. When undergoing a surgical procedure myself, one of the things my doctor told me was, and this is when I knew I had the right doctor, she said, "Your attitude is very important in this whole thing." In other words, she gave it back to me. It is my body, it is my choice whether I get swallowed up by this experience or whether I take charge. I may not get the end result I want, but I can work with that. In other words, some people do not get healed. For lack of a better word, they are "handicapped," or injured, and they have to then deal with that. You *can* roll over and die, but typically, that doesn't serve you. It's very important, then, that you take charge, and you redefine yourself. One thing I haven't talked about yet is balance. Balance is really important. Sometimes when I see patients who are depressed, or obsessive, or anxiety-ridden, they're out of balance. They've lost their friends, their families, their interests, and as I've said, their whole focus is now on their injury or pain. That is not life. We do things in balance. We sleep for a period of time in order for us to wake and be active for a period of time, and then we have to sleep again, because that's the balance of life. When something ends in your life, if you are injured, for example, and you now have to end your work or your hobby, it's important that your whole self isn't defined by that work or hobby—that there are other aspects of your like which *also* define you. And that you feel the confidence to develop something else which can also define you, something that maybe you haven't had the time to work on. Maybe it's your creative side. "Well, no, but I have to make money." There are *many* ways to make money! We all have the capability to make productive choices. That doesn't come from a pill. That comes from inside yourself. One of my favorite sayings is "No matter where you go, there you are." Another is "Limits exist only in your mind."

TC: Can you talk about the relationship between stress and pain?

LRC: There is a cycle in the body that occurs where there is pain, which creates tension, which creates muscle tension, which creates anxiety, which creates more pain. And then you go through it again and again. In the end it creates exhaustion for the whole body. This also can occur in your mind, as well—we call it "anticipatory anxiety," anticipating feeling the pain. This can lead to whole-body pain. A patient will now say [in describing symptoms], "Oh, well, now it's all over, it's *everywhere*. I never go without pain." They've gone through this cycle so much that now all they see is pain.

TC: Dr. Haack-Rogers, I've spoken with so many people who've had to change careers or give up a favorite hobby in order to heal from a repetitive strain injury. There's no question this can be devastating. We sometimes derive our sense of self from our occupation. How do we deal with these types of changes and redefine ourselves?

LRC: Again, it is important that people develop a vision for themselves and of themselves, and that they work on defining themselves, their goals, their successes, and what success means to them. Counseling can help to bring that into reality. If a person were to say, "I'd consider myself a success if I were to make a million dollars," I would challenge them and say, "Do you think that Mother Theresa is a success?" I don't know one person who would say no. And yet, she doesn't have a million dollars. It goes back into a larger picture and a larger balance, and having a clear, reality-based vision for yourself. It's important to make sure that these definitions are well within your capabilities, matching your talents with your physical state. Sometimes, people do less than they are capable of because they are afraid. Others do more than they should, and they re-injure themselves. Check and review your goals with your medical doctor, your counselor, or even your boss. Make sure that your level of activity is appropriate. Share your list of goals and visions with your family and friends. People don't know you unless you express to them who you are and what you'd like, but they can generally do a pretty good job of supporting you when your needs and goals have been clearly communicated. If you see yourself as a victim, you will be a victim. We only victimize ourselves.

You can also make verbal affirmations to yourself to help strengthen your mental attitude:

- "I know I can do this today."
- "I feel really good about myself."
- "I feel strength in my body."
- "I feel my pain reduced."

Be prepared for setbacks. What I mean by "prepared" is just to know that these occur. Setbacks are learning experiences, rather than failures. We all slip at times, no matter what we engage in. This is part of the learning process. Keep your mind open to learning new things, such as aspects of yourself and your body. Don't see a setback as pushing you back to step one; that's not true at all.

Finally, don't let others define who you are and what you need. Your boss or your spouse might tell you what you should be doing, but it's important to get clear on what your vision is. Define yourself first—define your goals, what it means for you to be successful.

To contact Dr. Linda Haack-Rogers personally, write or call:

16935 West Bernardo Drive, Suite 108A
San Diego, CA 92127
(619) 451-0771

Stress is universal, but the effective management of stress is highly individual. Fortunately, there is no shortage in our society of stress reduction books, videos, workshops, and gurus. It's important not to take stress lightly as it relates to your health. Whether you choose meditation, exercise, a support group, talking with a mental health professional, joining a church, or screaming into a pillow, do explore some of the many possible ways to prevent stress from taking its toll on your physical health. Total health is a combination of physical, mental, emotional, and spiritual wellness. Don't neglect any part!

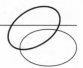

CHAPTER SEVEN

Prevention and Self-Help

When working with new employees on proper job habits and injury prevention, the first thing I stress is this: *you don't have to get it!* Carpal Tunnel Syndrome and other related injuries are not necessarily an inevitable part of using your hands a lot. However, it does require effort and commitment on your part to ensure healthy arms and hands, and that's what this chapter is about. Just like a dancer or a professional athlete, you must actively prepare your body to perform with minimal risk of injury.

Until recently, many people were unaware of what this syndrome is called. They may have attributed their symptoms to overwork, stress, tension, or assumed it was a natural part of their particular profession. Unfortunately, not all physicians and health care professionals are familiar enough with overuse injuries to be able to identify the cause and appropriate treatment. Patients have been told to put up with it, to stop what they are doing, or to wait until it worsens enough to warrant treatment. Even now, rarely is a patient given accurate, up-to-date information on the wide variety of options available in conservative care. And in some cases the patient's condition deteriorates to the point where conservative treatment programs are no longer effective, and complete immobilization of the hands and arms and/or surgery are the only alternatives.

It's not unusual to feel helpless when faced with a chronic condition that requires many lifestyle changes and a potentially long course of treatment. The good news is that there are steps you can take now to prevent the symptoms of repetitive strain injury from occurring or worsening. And if you are in the moderate to severe stages of CTS, it's not too late to learn some new techniques for taking care of yourself at home to prevent further damage and help to relieve the pain or numbness you may be experiencing. These suggestions are not a substitute for professional medical care when it is needed. Discuss what you've learned with your care provider, and with her approval, experiment with some of the ideas offered here until you find the unique combination that works for you.

Self-Testing

If you suspect you may be developing Carpal Tunnel Syndrome, you can check your own arms and hands to see if any problems are developing. One simple test is to simply make the "A-OK" sign with each hand—a circle with the thumb and forefinger. Ask a friend to try to separate the fingers. If the thumb and forefinger separate easily, you may have a loss of muscle strength or problem with the nerve.

The previously described Phalen's and Tinel's tests can be done regularly at home. (see Chapter Three, Figures 9 and 10).

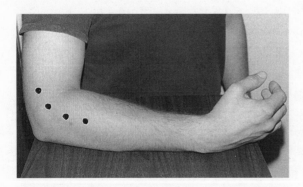

Figure 20. Potential trigger points along the elbow

You can also check points along the elbow [Figure 20], on the outside and inside of the arm, for pain and swelling. Tenderness in these areas suggests that the muscles in the arms may be working excessively.

Stiffness, tightness, pain, and/or restricted movement from the neck down into the upper shoulders or arms can be a warning that the arms and hands may eventually develop some problems. These muscles should be treated and the joints in the neck examined to ensure maximum mobility and to reduce the stiffness and pain.

Nutrition

You met Dr. Ray Wunderlich, Jr. in Chapter Five. In his work with CTS patients Dr. Wunderlich, who specializes in nutrition and preventative medicine, addresses the connection between conditions like CTS and nutrition, and the importance of providing the body with the "raw materials" it needs for maintenance and repair. Undernourishment, yeast overgrowth, food allergies, faulty digestion, and reaction to toxins are some of the factors that may weaken the body or intensify the trauma of constant repetitive movements.

If your diet includes a high percentage of processed, packaged foods, sugar, salt (which can cause water retention), soft drinks, fat, etc., it's time to take a hard look at your eating habits and replace unhealthy foods with a new, improved diet, emphasizing a variety of whole, natural foods and designed to *support* your body rather than deplete its resources. This was one of the hardest changes for me to make. Ice, splints, rest, even surgery—nothing compared to cutting down on sugar and especially salt in my diet. My four food groups were sugar, salt, fat, and chocolate! But I eventually realized that all the doctors and treatments in the world were not going to help me unless I started taking care of myself from the inside out. I cut out the junk (well, most of it), started walking every day, and got on a medically sensible program of nutritional supplements. Sure enough, my symptoms got better—it was the extra push I needed to close the gap between where I was and where I wanted to be physically.

Don't expect miracles. Strive for slow and steady improvements. You may even feel worse at first as your body rids itself of built-up toxins and waste. Treat yourself to an ice cream sundae once in a while—total deprivation is misery and not necessary for most people.

Another factor to consider is **sugar**—high levels of refined sugar in the diet have been shown to reduce the body's overall ability to fight off inflammation, colds, allergies, etc. Dr. Michael Madden, in his injury prevention workshops, advises patients that a diet heavy in processed sugar creates stress on the pancreas and the adrenal glands, exhausting the body's own natural ability to reduce inflammation and fight infection. Avoid sugar completely when inflammation is present, and reduce your regular intake on a daily basis. Get into the habit of reaching for a piece of fruit instead of a doughnut or a candy bar. You may notice a big difference not only in your hands and arms, but in your energy level, moods, and immune system.

Vitamins and Minerals

Studies have shown that in some cases a deficiency of **vitamin B6** may play a role in the development of Carpal Tunnel Syndrome (see Appendix B, "Articles"). Fifty to one hundred mg. per day of B6, taken with a complete B-complex supplement, improves symptoms considerably for many patients. B6 is also a natural diuretic, relieving water retention which can worsen symptoms (water retention is one explanation for the increased pain and tingling some women experience premenstrually and during pregnancy). Birth control pills can deplete the body's supply of B6, so if you are on the pill and experiencing symptoms of CTS, consider supplementing your diet with B6.

Vitamin B6 supplements should be taken with care—ironically, excessive amounts can cause the very symptoms you are trying to relieve. I spoke with a woman who told me she had tried B6 but it hadn't worked; in fact, she was worse now than before. The pain and numbness in her hands, wrists, and now *legs* were severe. When I asked her how much B6 she was taking each day, she replied "800 milligrams," or *eight times* the recommended dose! Her family doctor had approved, telling her it was "impossible to overdose on B vitamins." Under a different doctor's care, she gradually lowered the dosage, and the last time she contacted me she had begun to get some of the feeling back in her fingers. Was it the B6? It's hard to say for sure, but it's certainly an example to the rest of us to use care when putting *anything* into our bodies, whether it is medication, herbal or homeopathic remedies, or even vitamin supplements. More is not necessarily better!

Many of us can benefit from certain supplements, particularly when our diets are not all they should be. However, standing in the store and staring at the arrays of vitamins, minerals, herbs, capsules, and shakes is enough to make most of us give up. It would take a degree in chemistry to understand most labels. But do take the time to learn the basics of what effects vitamins, minerals, and herbs can have on your body. Talk to health care professionals and read up on the many products available today. And again, stay away from hard-core fads—as with exercise, diet, and therapeutic programs, a sensible, middle-of-the-road approach is usually safest. There are some wonderful products on the market, and some which are not so wonderful. Look for quality ingredients and production. Learn about which supplements are designed to be utilized efficiently by the body and which ones are a waste of your money. Calcium supplements, for example, vary widely in their effectiveness.

The best line of products I've found so far is produced by Body Wise International, Inc., located in Carlsbad, California. Body Wise offers a complete system of scientifically advanced nutritional products manufactured under pharmaceutical-caliber conditions. I was impressed not only by the quality and effectiveness of the products themselves, but also by the effort the company puts into consumer education. More information on Body Wise International can be found in Appendix C.

More Suggestions for Self-Help

Every practitioner I spoke with, regardless of specialty, recommended *rest* from aggravating activities and modification of daily habits to allow the injured nerve to heal. Regular breaks during any activity involving the hands and arms is often enough to halt the problem before it worsens. It's as simple as taking a break. Be aware of your own physical limitations when performing any task requiring repetitive movement. Are you becoming fatigued or

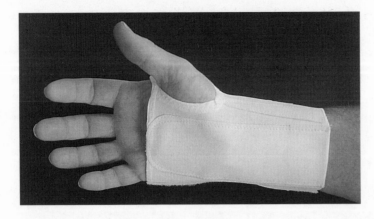

Figure 21. Wrist splint

stiffening up? Have your hands or neck been in an awkward position for a prolonged period of time? Most people need to take a short break after every twenty to forty minutes of continuous activity to stretch, walk around, or just relax the hands and arms. And if you can elevate the arm, perhaps propping it up on a cushion for a few minutes, all the better.

Immobilization through the use of **wrist splints,** which hold the wrist in a non-flexed position [Figure 21] are recommended in some cases. The splint should fit well but not so tight that circulation is impaired. A too-tight splint can do more harm than good. It should *limit* range of movement, but not prevent it entirely. You should be able to move the wrist slightly (about ten percent of your normal range of motion) while wearing the splint. Wrist splints are helpful for some people; however, splints should not be seen as a permanent fix. In fact, splints are not as universally recommended as they were a few years ago. They can effectively keep the wrist in a neutral position, particularly if you sleep with your hands in an awkward position. But when symptoms begin to subside, wean away from the splints and develop a program of exercise to allow you to regain function and mobility in the arms. And if your wrist splints don't provide any relief or they cause your symptoms to worsen, by all means talk to your health care practitioner.

A *forearm brace* can be very effective in relieving pain in the elbow and forearm. These simple bands are often used for "tennis elbow," and can be purchased in most drug or medical supply stores for around $5 to $10. As with the wrist splint, do not tighten the forearm brace so much that you cut off circulation to your hand. It should fit snugly but comfortably [Figure 22].

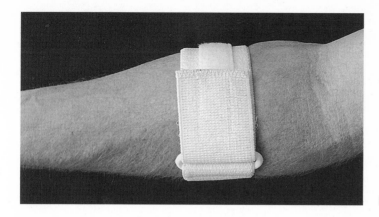

Figure 22. Forearm brace

The use of *ice packs* can help to reduce inflammation. Apply the pack to the affected areas, right on the hand, wrist or elbow if needed, throughout the day for 10- to 15-minute periods. You can even massage the injured area with the ice pack for extra relief. If you experience discomfort, discontinue use. Don't have an ice pack? A baggie full of frozen popcorn (unpopped, of course) or peas works just as well in an emergency.

The application of *moist heat,* particularly to the neck and shoulder areas, can help to relax tight muscles. Wet a towel with hot water (*comfortably* hot—don't burn yourself), wring it out well, wrap it around a hot water bottle, and lie down on your back so that your neck and shoulders are resting on the towel. Relax for 10-15 minutes. A regular heating pad can feel good as well, but moist heat is more penetrating and its effects longer-lasting.

Ice vs. Heat

When should you apply heat to an injury, and when is ice the best choice? Ice is used when there is inflammation to prevent or reduce swelling, particularly in the acute stages. The application of cold constricts blood vessels in the area and prevents them from bleeding. Heat *draws* blood to an injured area and the increased circulation assists in the body's attempts to heal itself. Heat works best after the acute stage has passed, rather than immediately after an injury or when inflammation is present, when it could actually worsen swelling.

Handeze Gloves

During the course of writing two books on repetitive strain injuries I've been sent a number of products, videos, and books designed to relieve the pain and tingling of RSIs, ranging from effective to potentially dangerous. I consider myself fairly skeptical, so my initial response was cautious when I received a thick packet full of products and patient/practitioner testimonials from Therapeutic Appliance Group, the company which manufactures a product known as Handeze Gloves. The claims were dramatic. Court reporters, medical transcriptionists, professional musicians, sign language instructors, even physicians reported not only symptom relief but the ability to return to previous activity levels without strain. A. Robert Mailloux of the Therapeutic Appliance Group included several samples for me to try, and because I was in a full-blown flareup of symptoms in both hands from long hours at the keyboard, I slipped on a pair of the Musician's Practice and Warm-Up Gloves and sat down at the computer.

Within twenty minutes, I was a new convert. The gloves retain body heat, raising the temperature in the wrist, hand, and fingers—a real benefit for me because my hands are usually cold, which invariably worsens my symptoms. The specially-treated Lycra material provides support and a feeling similar to massage, but without a feeling of restriction. I was able to type easily while wearing the gloves. The packet also included a newer product: Wrist-Mate wrist supports for those who require additional support at the wrist. The gloves are available in a variety of styles and colors, and sizing is important. When I tried a size just slightly too large, the effects were minimal. Therapeutic Appliance Group stresses the need for proper sizing and will assist customers in determining their correct size. I found this product far more comfortable and effective than splints, and the effects lasted even after I removed the gloves. This is a product definitely worth a second look—affordable (around $20), practical, and effective. Check Appendix C for more information about Handeze Gloves and the Therapeutic Appliance Group.

There are plenty of choices today if you'd like to purchase a cold or hot pack, including microwavable heat wraps, packs that slip inside a sleeve or cervical collar, even mittens made of spandex material containing a gel which can be activated in a microwave, conventional oven, or freezer.

Massage is extremely useful in relaxing tight and sometimes spasmed muscles in the arm, shoulders, neck and middle back. Your best bet is a professional massage therapist as discussed in Chapter Five, preferably one knowledgable about repetitive stress injuries. You can also employ self-massage, especially helpful when directed to the inner and outer forearm and the neck. In a pinch, an electric massager can help to relax sore, tight muscles, and can allow you to work on hard-to-reach areas like the upper back. I've heard of offices with a high rate of overuse injuries (data entry operators, for example) who began keeping an electric massager or two in a convenient place in the office for workers to use during break times. One of the best is Conair's Sonassage Sonic Pain Reliever, which comes with a variety of attachments, including one specially designed for the hand and fingers. Massage is *not* recommended when there is a lot of inflammation and pain present, when deep massage could actually do more harm than good.

Home treatment will help to ensure maximum neck mobility. If your neck has certain structural problems that affect your injury, cervical exercises (see Chapter Nine), home traction devices (you'll need a doctor's recommendation for this), and cervical pillows can all help you maintain your health on a daily basis. Remember to first have a physician check for hereditary bone abnormalities, osteoarthritis, and muscle, ligament, or disk damage from accidents.

Be sure to address any underlying systemic disease and take steps to ***improve your physical condition.*** If your general health is poor or your symptoms are worsened by any of the conditions discussed in Chapter One, begin taking care of yourself now. Take a hard look at your life. How is your diet? Do you smoke or use drugs? Do you get some form of regular exercise appropriate to your fitness level? What about the amount of stress in your life? See a physician for a complete physical exam and discuss any health concerns you may have.

Topical application of homeopathic remedies, ginger soaks/compresses (see below) or salves like Tiger Balm, Sunbreeze®, or Mineral Ice® provide

---

Ginger compress

Grate fresh ginger and wrap in a cloth. Squeeze the cloth so the juice drips down into a pot of hot water, then dip a hand towel into the ginger water. Wring out, then apply hot (but not scalding) to the injured area. Cover with a dry towel to retain heat. Replace every three to five minutes.

---

temporary relief. They feel good, and sometimes at the end of the day a gentle massage with one of these topical ointments can help you relax tired, tense muscles.

A **paraffin bath** is a warm mixture of paraffin wax (available in medical and/or beauty supply stores) and mineral oil—four parts wax to one part oil. The wax and oil are melted down, and the hand is dipped repeatedly into the mixture, building up layers of paraffin. The heat deeply penetrates into the muscles and tendons, and has been found to help with arthritic pain and stiffness. Wrap the paraffin-coated hand in a warm, moist towel and allow the heat to penetrate the hand for fifteen to twenty minutes. Then peel away the wax, and massage and gently stretch and exercise the hand. You can melt the wax yourself (carefully!) on the stove over low heat, or purchase a special heating unit designed especially for paraffin baths. Either way, use caution to avoid being burned by a too-hot mixture. I have a paraffin bath unit and use it regularly, and it always feels great and relieves stiffness—definitely worth the high price I paid for it! Remember, when there is inflammation present it is preferable to apply ice to an injury rather than heat.

Self-Help Suggestions from Readers

Chances are, whether you are in the beginning stages of Carpal Tunnel Syndrome or have just completed a treatment program, your injury has become a part of your life. We use our hands innumerable times each day. If you are in pain, you have a constant reminder. If you have recovered, you've probably made permanent changes in your way of life to help ensure that you never become injured again.

"I use an inflatable lumbar roll, rather than the standard kind. It lets me adjust the amount of support depending on the chair I'm in."

"I wear Isotoner® gloves, which seem to keep my hands extra warm while allowing freedom of movement." [Note: Isotoner® also makes a therapeutic glove especially for control of swelling, in various styles including a fingerless glove. See Smith & Nephew Rolyan ordering info in Appendix C]

"I fill up one side of my double sink with warm water, the other with cold, then alternate soaking my hands for five to ten minutes each."

"When I purchased my new car, I made sure it had an automatic transmission and power steering for less wear and tear on my hands."

"Allow plenty of time for rest in between concentrated work hours. Know your limits and be assertive in not exceeding them."

"It sounds crazy, but I lie down on a tennis ball and roll around. It gets the kinks out of my back."

"I exercise and stretch my whole body in the mornings. I try to release the tension building in my neck or back during each break."

"My schedule is jam-packed from morning till night, but when I feel tense in the evening I steal a few minutes under a hot shower, with my shower massage attachment turned on high to loosen up my shoulders and neck."

"I learned how to ask for help."

Check the final chapter of this book for more thoughts and suggestions from fellow CTS/RSI patients.

Keeping a Journal

It is helpful for both you and your doctor if you keep track of your symptoms on a daily basis, including which activities make you feel better or worse. Habits, work duties, diet, exercise, menstruation—all can have a great deal of influence on your symptoms.

Keeping a daily journal can help you see patterns developing, and whether you are improving or going downhill. Day-to-day changes can seem slow, even going backwards at times, so a journal kept over a long period can show slow but steady changes.

Start out by assigning a numerical value from 0 to 10 to the pain levels in your hands, wrists, arms, neck, and/or back. (If you are experiencing numbness, tingling, weakness, etc., record those levels, too.) Use 10 to indicate the very worst pain, and 1 as completely pain-free.

Improvements can be noted by a decrease in the numbers or the fact that it begins to take longer before symptoms arise. For example, suppose your wrist initially began to hurt at a level of 7 after ten minutes of typing. After two weeks of treatment it may still hurt, but now it takes thirty minutes before you are at the same level of 7.

Overuse injuries are not only caused by repetitive motion at work. Many people engage in hobbies that involve the hands—crafts, drawing, sewing, carpentry, knitting, operating a computer, or sporting activities. It is important to note whether your hands are being overused, hyperextended, or hyperflexed in these non-work related activities as well, and apply what you've learned to the activities of your everyday life.

Keep a record of how your diet affects your symptoms. Do you notice an increase in pain and numbness after a meal high in salt? Do you feel sluggish a few hours after eating a candy bar? Do vitamin B supplements help?

I have provided a sample weekly chart to assist you in keeping track of your treatment and symptoms. Feel free to make copies or revise it in any way that works best for you.

Sample Journal

Keeping a journal: Recording your daily habits and symptoms on a chart like this one will help you keep track of your progress as you go through your treatment plan. This is valuable information for your physician as well.

Learning about the many ways you can take care of yourself is empowering. It is unrealistic, and even unwise in some cases, to believe we can diagnose and treat all repetitive strain injuries by ourselves. A trained health care professional can assist you in determining the nature and severity of your injuries, and make recommendations about your treatment program. The ideas in this chapter are here to supplement that care and to assist you in functioning as a partner with your doctor.

Week of			
Monday	Tuesday	Wednesday	Thursday
Treatment: Symptoms:	Treatment: Symptoms:	Treatment: Symptoms:	Treatmen:; Symptoms:
Friday	Saturday	Sunday	Notes
Treatment: Symptoms:	Treatment: Symptoms:	Treatment: Symptoms:	

Treatment: list any medications, therapy (massage, manipulation, physical therapy), self-help (ice, rest, splints, warm-up/stretching, stress reduction), changes in diet, etc.

Symptoms: on a scale of 1-10, with 10 being the worst pain and 1 the least, rate any symptoms you experience each day. Specify whether you feel pain, numbness, tingling, or weakness.

Make a special note on days you use your arms and hands a lot, so you can see how extra activity affects your symptoms.

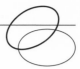

CHAPTER EIGHT

Repetitive Strain Injuries in the Workplace

Many of us with repetitive strain injury got that way on the job. This is not intended to be an indictment of employers in general—I truly believe that most employers are as taken aback by the epidemic of overuse injuries as those of us who are diagnosed with them, and I know many supervisors and employers who sincerely want to help their employees prevent injuries. There are also, however, horror stories of injured employees enduring harassment or even losing their jobs due to these injuries. Several of you have written to me describing how you simply work with the pain, knowing your conditions are worsening day by day but frightened to do anything about it. A number of people diagnosed with work-related repetitive strain injuries who contributed their personal stories to Chapter Ten asked that their names be withheld in order to avoid repercussions on the job.

This chapter is designed to provide you with answers to some of the most common questions regarding work-related injuries, and ideally to give you some support as well as options you may not have considered for making your work environment a healthier place.

The Americans with Disabilities Act

At this writing, the Americans with Disabilities Act (ADA)is in effect for all employers with fifteen or more employees. The ADA prohibits discrimination on the basis of disability as long as the person is qualified to perform the *essential functions* of the job, with or without a *reasonable accommodation*, if it would not impose an undue hardship on the operation of the employer's business.

What Do You Mean by "Essential Functions"?

The essential functions of a job are the duties that are most fundamental to the performance of the job. For a secretary, the essential functions of the job may include typing, filing, answering and routing phone calls, and distributing the mail.

What is a Reasonable Accommodation?

A reasonable accommodation is some modification in the job's tasks or the work environment which will allow the qualified employee with a disability to perform the essential functions of the job.

If your disability is interfering with your job, the first thing to do is perform a job analysis. What really are the essential functions of the job? What percentage of time do you spend on each? What accommodations could be made that would help you work more productively? Get a copy of your job description to help you identify key duties.

Next, see your physician to document your condition and ask for his feedback in your job analysis. In his opinion, what modifications in your job duties would allow you to work without worsening your symptoms?

Now your background work is complete, and you're ready to approach your employer to discuss some ideas for reasonable accommodations. Now is not the time to be accusing or defensive. Your goal should be a "win-win" outcome, where both you and your employer come away satisfied, with a better understanding of the other's needs. I know some of you are rolling your eyes at this point—"Not my boss . . . never in a million years!" It's unrealistic to assume every employer will display a willingness to accommodate an injured worker. But by preparing yourself in advance, your chances of a satisfactory outcome are increased.

Be ready with some suggestions for ways your duties, schedule, or work environment could be modified to allow you to perform the essential functions of your job while still protecting your health. Show your employer that you have given some thought to ways you can remain a productive member of the work team. Emphasize your *capabilities,* not your limitations.

Here are a few ideas to help you get started:

- Would the purchase of some ergonomic equipment allow you to perform repetitive tasks more easily?
- Could you juggle job duties with other staff members? For example, if another worker's job primarily involves answering phones and filing and you spend all day keyboarding, could the two of you switch duties periodically?
- Would a reduction in work hours help, or even working at home a couple of days a week?

I'm an employer and I'm concerned about the rise in work-related injuries. What can I do to protect myself and my workers?

Evaluate: Review each position and its essential functions. Take a good look at each employee's workstation. Bring in an ergonomics consultant if necessary to help you get a complete understanding of each employee's job.

Communicate: Talk to your employees. Your workers can often be your best source of ideas to assist you in finding the balance between productivity and safety. Express your needs and take a team approach to designing a healthy and efficient system.

Educate: Yourself and your employees—how do these injuries occur and what can be done to prevent them? Departments like Risk Management, Human Resources, and Employee Benefits can be a source of up-to-date information for employees on healthy work habits, exercise, diet, and other topics related to safety and health.

Workers' Compensation

Workers' Compensation is an insurance program mandated by federal and states governments requiring employers to cover lost wages and medical expenses for employees who are injured on the job. Workers' Compensation laws help to protect employees who are injured or disabled on the job, eliminating the need for costly litigation. With few exceptions, nearly every employee is covered by Workers' Compensation.

The first step is to report promptly *any* injury to your immediate supervisor. You will be asked to complete a claim form describing the injury. In many states you are required initially to see the doctor who represents your employer's Workers' Compensation insurance company, then after a specified time (usually thirty days), you can choose the health care provider of your choice. The choice of health care provider is even more significant when Workers' Compensation is involved—typically these insurance companies discourage changing doctors more than once or twice, and only with a compelling reason.

Workers' Compensation in California recognizes two broad categories of injuries related to employment. Many injuries that occur on the job are caused by *specific* accidents, like a cut finger or a fall. *Cumulative trauma* is somewhat more complicated—it may be hard to pinpoint the exact date of injury, for example, if you are required to provide that information on a claim form. Repetitive strain injuries are not the only claims filed due to injuries caused by continuous trauma. For example, workers exposed to hazardous materials, such as asbestos, also suffer the cumulative effects of an unsafe working environment.

Designating Your Own Physician

You may, in many states, file a special form with your employer which allows you to see your own physician in the event of an injury at work, rather than a doctor selected by your employer or Workers' Compensation insurance carrier. Ask your Human Resources department or Benefits office if this is an option for you.

Worker's Compensation laws are complex and oftentimes confusing. Not every claimant hires an attorney, however, many of the patients I interviewed expressed their relief in hiring a professional to negotiate a settlement, assist in selecting a doctor, examine medical reports, and act as a go-between between the claimant and the insurance company. Few claimants have the expertise of a Workers' Compensation claims adjuster, and it is easy to become overwhelmed by the system. Sometimes, professional assistance is needed. Attorneys don't work for free; expect to pay a fee of around 12-15% of your final settlement award to your attorney. From personal experience, it can be worth every penny.

Most injuries that occur on the job are caused by accidents, like a cut finger or a fall. Injuries due to continuous trauma are somewhat more complicated—it may be hard to pinpoint the exact date of injury, for example, if you are required to provide that information on a claim form. Repetitive strain injuries are not the only work-related disorders arising from cumulative trauma. Continued exposure to hazardous materials, such as asbestos, can lead to the degradation of an employee's health.

Workers' Compensation can reimburse you for medical costs, lost wages, permanent disability, rehabilitation services, and even vocational training to prepare you for a different occupation. Benefits vary from state to state. For example, in California workers suffering from Carpal Tunnel Syndrome are protected under the state's compensation program, while a February 1996 decision by the state Supreme Court in Virginia ruled that employees who develop CTS are not eligible to collect Workers' Compensation benefits, even with verification from a physician that the injury is work-related. For information on Workers' Compensation in your state, call the nearest office of the State Division of Workers' Compensation. They can help you understand your rights and answer any questions you have. If you belong to a union, your representative should be able to advise you as well. And, if none of these avenues are satisfactory, it may be necessary to hire an attorney to handle your claim for you.

If the injury interferes with your work but is not work-related (directly caused by the duties of your job), you may be eligible for some kind of state disability if you need time off to recover. Check with your employer's benefits office. If your injury is not work-related, your private medical insurance

---

What is OSHA?

In 1970, the Occupational Safety and Health Act was passed to assure safe working conditions for working men and women. OSHA (the Occupational Safety and Health Administration) assists state and federal governments in the enforcing the standards set forth in the Occupational Safety and Health Act, such as providing research in the field of occupational safety, training programs, site inspections, and consultation services.

---

may cover some of the costs of medical treatment. Many insurance companies will now also cover chiropractic care and acupuncture. Check your policy to find out what services are covered.

Workers' Compensation can be an expensive solution for your employer and his insurance carrier. If several of your co-workers are experiencing problems similar to yours, it may be time to sit down and make some changes—whether in each worker's workstation, in the scheduling of each shift, or in establishing a program to educate workers who are at risk. Often these kinds of changes cost much less in the long run than absences, surgeries, vocational rehabilitation, and retraining new personnel.

Some final suggestions if you must file a Workers' Compensation claim:

- *Be honest.* Filing a false claim is a felony in California, subject to a fine of up to $50,000 or up to five years in prison. You'll be interviewed by the insurance company and their staff doctors. You may even need to give a deposition or be videotaped. Your previous medical history will be open for review by everyone involved in your case. Exaggerating your symptoms or making fraudulent statements can not only have serious consequences for you, but every false claim makes it that much harder for legitimate cases to proceed through the system.
- *Report any injury promptly.* Most states have a time limit during which you can file a claim for a work-related injury. Be sure all paperwork is filed accurately and in a timely manner. Telling your employer is the first step, but you must also file an official claim with your state's Workers' Compensation office.

- ***Be an active participant in your case.*** Keep records—a journal is a good way to keep track of events, symptoms, and conversations with your employer and the insurance company. Learn about your state's laws and what benefits you are entitled to receive. Ask questions.
- ***Obtain the best medical care you can.*** What this means is, as I've mentioned in previous chapters, choose a physician with your best interests at heart. Health care professionals can sometimes get caught on one side of the fence or another in Workers' Compensation wars. Your doctor's primary concern should be helping you get well. Do your homework before designating a physician to handle your care, since Workers' Compensation insurance carriers, understandably, frown on hopping from doctor to doctor.

Ergonomics

Observe an injured worker on the job, and chances are you'll spot a problem with posture and/or the physical layout of the workstation. With some retraining and simple improvements in the workplace, injuries can be decreased and even prevented.

Ergonomics is a big word for a simple concept: it basically refers to the idea of creating a work environment that promotes physical health and comfort while optimizing job performance. Overuse injuries are at epidemic levels in the workplace. Employers are discovering that it is actually more cost-effective to make the initial investment in furniture and equipment designed to *prevent* physical stresses than to deal with the problem of work-related injuries down the line.

The epidemic numbers of repetitive strain injuries reported by the Bureau of Labor Statistics naturally has led many businesses to jump on the ergonomic bandwagon. Currently, the market is flooded with devices and furniture labeled "ergonomic," but are they? People suffering from RSIs, eager for relief and the promise of pain-free wrists, plunked down hundreds of dollars for ergonomic chairs with enough levers and gears to *cause* Carpal Tunnel Syndrome, footrests that they had to strain to reach, or rock-hard wrist rests in designer colors that left indentations on their wrists. Just as in selection of health care, consumerism is coming into play in the field of ergonomics. Support groups, publications, and resources like the RSI Electronic Newsletter are weeding through the vast array of products out there and reporting back to fellow sufferers as to what works and what doesn't.

The ultimate decision rests with you, the consumer. When choosing a piece of office furniture or a product designed to help alleviate the physical stresses associated with long hours at the computer, ask around. Get product brochures, visit a showroom, and talk with your health care professional or an ergonomics specialist (preferably one without his or her *own* product to sell you!). Sit in that chair, adjust those levers, pound that adjustable keyboard. Our bodies are built differently, and you'll want to try out a variety of products until you find the right fit for you.

This chapter will help you make some important (and in some cases, expensive) decisions about redesigning your work space to optimize your physical capabilities. And remember, these are just guidelines. The more you learn and the more questions you ask, the better equipped you'll be to make smart choices in office design.

Let's take a look at a typical work environment to identify some potential problem areas.

The Right Chair

When you consider how many hours most of us spend sitting at sedentary desk jobs, it's no wonder our backs hurt! Many injuries start with poorly designed seating. An uncomfortable chair leads to postural problems, which in turn throw off the alignment of the spine and impair nerve function to the arms and hands. So, let's start with chair design. The ideal chair should be adjustable to a height that is comfortable for you—sixteen to twenty inches is best. Your weight should be forward and your arms at desk height. Both feet should rest flat on the floor; if they don't reach, use a footrest. Hips and knees should be at the same height to reduce stress on the legs. The lower back needs support, whether from the chair itself or through the use of a lumbar cushion or rolled-up towel. The chair should be easily adjustable.

Even the best chair won't help if you slump or slouch. Keep your spine and head upright, and prevent slouching by sitting *back* into the chair. That $500 chair is terrific while you are at work, but remember you sit at home, in the car, and elsewhere, too, and be kind to your back wherever you are. Do everything you can to avoid the "couch potato" lifestyle. If you like to unwind in front of the television in the evening, hit the floor and do your stretches while you watch your favorite show. Give the same consideration to your home furnishings, especially your sofa and mattress, as you do your work environment. When my husband and I were shopping recently for a new sofa and loveseat, we were dismayed at the "mushy" feel of most of the sofas we tested. Invariably we would sink down in a sea of overstuffed cushions, our knees nearly shoulder-level. Getting up was a strain, too. We finally found a firm set with plenty of back support and we're glad we took the time to shop with our spines in mind!

One last, but important, note about sitting. *Don't do it all day long!* Get up and walk around. Give your circulation a chance to get moving again. Alternate duties you spend sitting down with those you can do in a standing position. Stretch, brace yourself against a wall and do a couple of the stretches in Chapter Nine, or take a short walk around the building.

The "Inflammation Superhighway"—Computers

Spending long hours at a computer can take its toll on your hands, wrists, and neck, leading to strain and injury. Modern technology has given us word processors and computers able to handle the fastest keystrokes we can dish out. No longer do we have to pause to push a carriage return, manually correct a mistake, or change paper. Unfortunately, all the little details that went along with those old-fashioned typewriters might have helped some of us to avoid the injuries that come from hours of keyboarding, frozen in one position, with machines built to handle far more speed and volume than we can physically put out. The problem is our bodies are the same as they've always been, and keeping up with our equipment, not to mention deadlines and quotas, can lead to injury. However, there are many simple things you can do to improve your workstation and create a more comfortable environment.

First, raise your computer monitor to around *eye level* to reduce strain on the neck. If you are bending your head down (or in any direction) to see the screen comfortably, you are putting excess strain on the cervical spine and the muscles of the neck, which have to work harder to support the head when it is displaced from its natural position. Strain leads to muscle spasm, and since the nerves originating in the cervical spine enervate the hand and arms, pain and numbness below the area of the spasm can result. To help you adjust your monitor to a better height, there are a variety of monitor stands available in any computer supply store, or you can simply place your monitor on a stack of phone books. Be sure the monitor is positioned directly in front of you, to avoid twisting to view your work. I've seen a few attractively designed computer stations advertised as "ergonomic," when the monitor shelf was placed off to the left or right, requiring an awkward twist of the neck to view the screen.

The same principle applies when working with documents. Use a document holder to keep your papers at approximately eye level and take pressure off your neck as you work. Do not crane or twist your neck to read the copy. If your copy holder sits off to the right of your monitor, simply begin alternating sides periodically through the day so that you are not spending an entire day looking toward the right.

Your neck should be positioned directly above your shoulders. It's often difficult for us to identify long-standing habits, such as forward head posturing or dropping the shoulders. Have a friend or co-worker observe you at work. Better yet, if you can, videotape yourself at your workstation to catch any postural problems.

Keep hands and wrists in a comfortable, relaxed, *neutral* position—not too high or held at an awkward angle. Your wrists should not be hyperflexed or -extended, nor should they be deviated (bent sideways) or allowed to rest on the edge of the desk, positions which all put undue stress on the muscles and tendons of the wrists. Forearms should be at right angles to the body, with the forearm parallel to the floor. Ninety degrees is the ideal angle for typing or data entry tasks. Some people appreciate the support of a padded armrest; however, for those with ulnar nerve impairment, resting the elbows can do more to impinge upon that nerve.

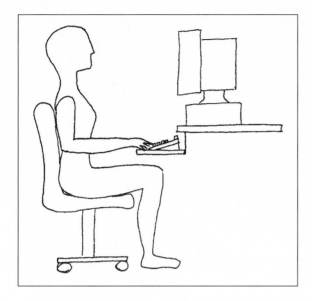

Figure 23. A well-designed workstation

The use of a wrist rest can be beneficial if you spend much time at a keyboard. Perhaps the term "wrist *rest*" is a misnomer—it can be too easy to end up pressing the wrist down onto the surface of the support, when actually wrist rests are better used as a reminder to keep the wrists in a neutral position. At no time should you lean on the wrist rest. When selecting a wrist rest for your keyboard, comfort should be your goal. I use an "Accu-Wrist" rest prescribed by my chiropractor, and its soft, padded design is an enormous help. I've recently seen a new *gel-filled* wrist rest for both the keyboard and the mouse which is a wonderful idea. Experiment to find what works best for you. Ask to try out the product before you buy. If you don't have a wrist rest, an idea you can try yourself is just to place a small, folded towel at the base of your keyboard, or even a folded piece of bubble wrap. A little extra support can go a long way in alleviating fatigue and tension.

We've discussed the basics for designing a healthy workstation. But as you'll soon see, there are far more options available in the ergonomic marketplace than chairs and keyboard monitors. Companies have come up with a wide selection of creative and helpful ideas for making your computer more "user-friendly."

Who's to Blame? Legal Issues and RSI

In early 1995 Nancy Urbanski, a former high school secretary now disabled by the effects of RSI, went to trial against Apple Computers and International Business Machines (IBM), claiming negligence on the part of the computer manufacturers. Thousands of lawsuits have been filed all over the country alleging that poor keyboard design and failure to adequately educate users about the possible health risks of computer use have led to injury and, in some cases, permanent disability. In 1994, Compaq Computer Corporation was found not liable for the injuries of a legal secretary who became injured after using one of the company's computers.

In Nancy Urbanski's case, on February 24, 1995, she reached a settlement with Apple Computers. The terms of the settlement were not disclosed; however, a spokesperson for Apple Computers indicated that their decision to settle was due to Apple's failure to supply Ms. Urbanski's attorneys with necessary company documents in a timely manner, rather than an admission of fault for the plaintiff's injuries. The case now proceeds with IBM as the sole defendant, and their attorneys expressed confidence in a favorable outcome.

The question of responsibility becomes even more complicated when we consider the role of computer manufacturers. What are the responsibilities of a company that designs and markets computers and keyboards? Should the blame lie with the supervisor who sets unreasonable standards in work production? What about the employee whose sedentary lifestyle or poor work habits lead to a greater vulnerability for injury? Where do we draw the line between true negligence on the part of a manufacturer and personal responsibility? There are no clear-cut answers. Each case is as individual as the people involved.

Some products to look for in your local computer supply store include:

* *Trackballs and mouse alternatives*—Many people complain that using a mouse creates more pain than typing. There are now a number of options available, including trackballs with foot pedals.

- *Ergonomic keyboards*—These range from a standard keyboard split into two separated keypads, to more user-friendly variations on the traditional QWERTY key layout, to the innovative DataHand, an "alternative" keyboard and mouse substitute which replaces conventional keys with padded palm supports and five-key finger modules.
- *Voice Recognition*—Imagine being able to use voice commands for many of the operations you now perform manually. There are a growing number of choices in adding voice recognition to your computer system. PowerSecretary, Dragon Dictate, VoiceType, IN3 PRO are a few of the titles available. Do a lot of research before adding voice recognition to your computer, as the prices can be pretty steep, and you want to be absolutely sure that the product meets your needs.
- *Keyboard platforms*—You can easily raise your keyboard to a comfortable height.
- *Adjustable wrist rests*—Available for your computer keyboard, ten-key adding machine, or mouse.
- *Gliding pads*—that attach to your keyboard, such as the Wrist Trolley™.

See Appendix C for information on these products.

You may need to do some rearranging of your workstation to achieve a setup that allows you to perform your duties and prevent injuries. Check your local computer or office supply store to ask about monitor stands, wrist rests, document holders, and other ideas to prevent repetitive motion injuries. There is even software available that, once installed in your computer, will remind you at set intervals to stretch or take a break! While writing my first book I frequently wore a Wrist Reminder™ by MicroComputer Accessories, Inc. Designed specifically to prevent or alleviate symptoms of overuse injuries, the Wrist Reminder is a comfortable wrist band with a plastic palm support, which provides support and limits wrist flexion while still allowing full range of motion of the fingers.

Writing by Hand

No question . . . if you have Carpal Tunnel Syndrome, writing by hand is a killer. During a flare-up of symptoms, it's all we can do to sign a check! If you write a lot by hand, purchase a few inexpensive soft pen/pencil grips to ease the strain on your fingers. Grab On Products makes comfortable foam grips in a size for nearly any need: pens, paint brushes, crochet hooks and knitting needles, drafting and gardening tools, brooms, even toothbrushes (see Appendix C for more information). I specified *soft* grips for a reason— there are a variety of grips on the market in all kinds of designs. The idea is to *relieve* pressure on the fingers and hands, and there are a few grips made of a fairly hard plastic which require nearly as much pressure to manipulate as if there were no grip used at all.

Most patients I've interviewed report that writing or drawing by hand for a prolonged period nearly always worsened symptoms considerably. Be sure to take frequent breaks to relax the hand and arm muscles if you are doing a lot of writing, and whenever possible avoid writing by hand while you are experiencing pain and numbness in your hand(s). A computer or typewriter may be easier for you to handle. And if you must write by hand, find a pen that writes easily without a lot of pressure.

Standing

Many of the same principles apply to those of you who work in a standing position. Keeping your spine in an aligned position [Figure 24] helps to alleviate strain. Move around, walk as much as you are able, alternate resting a leg on a footstool.

The following simple method can help to correct your standing posture: imagine a string running from the ceiling through the top of your head, down your back to your hips, pulling you up and helping you hold your head erect and spine straight. The shoulders should be back, and take care not to allow the hips to rotate out and back. Figure 25 illustrates a posture that is incorrect and may well lead to injuries.

Last, but not least, *slow down.* We all want to do our best on the job, producing the most work we can in the shortest period of time. Sometimes there is pressure from a supervisor to do it faster, faster, faster. With epidemic levels of repetitive strain injuries affecting most employers, it's clear that the increasing demands for more speed and more production are tak-

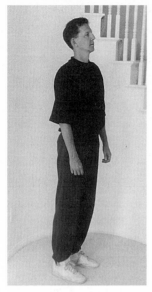   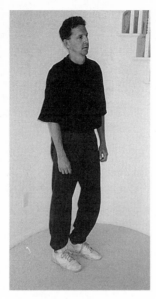

Figure 24. Correct posture   Figure 25. Incorrect posture

ing a toll on the nation's workforce. But we are not machines, and we must work within our own physical abilities. So give 100% to your employer, but make it reasonable and don't hurt yourself.

Talking with Gary Karp: The Onsight Solution

Controlling the rise of work-related injuries is often more than an employer can handle without expert assistance. Companies specializing in worksite evaluation and injury prevention are becoming increasingly visible as a way for employers to implement an individualized plan to reduce repetitive strain injuries in the workplace. Onsight, one such company based in San Francisco, offers ergonomic training, worksite evaluation, and a variety of services. Gary Karp, the company's founder and president, shares some thoughts with us.

TC: Gary, how did you get into this business?

GK: I am educated as an architect and have worked most of my professional life as a graphic artist in the presentation graphics business. I rose through the ranks as production manager, production system designer, computer graphics guru and trainer, and V.P. in charge of desktop services. The desktop work had me spending a lot of time at the keyboard, and with very poor ergonomics, though I didn't know it at the time. I continued to work with pain in my elbows and wrists for a year before going on disability and having a pretty complete experience of the Workers' Comp system. I dabbled in an array of treatments, from ultrasound to Chinese herbs, Feldenkrais and biofeedback. Myofascial release therapy has proven to be effective. I continue to be prone to flareups, have some pain every day, and have adapted in many ways, including a Maltron keyboard, voice dictation, and various hand-saving software solutions.

I had intended to start an education/communication company that helped people find their right relationship to computing. As a designer, trainer, manager, and entrepreneur I wanted to address the clear need people have to learn how to enjoy computing and tap its potential. Little did I know that my primary topic would become safety and ergonomics. Onsight Technology Education Services is my vocational rehabilitation plan. I began with development of a one-hour training session which had its trial presentations at support groups and a couple of freebies for potential clients.

TC: Tell me about what you do at Onsight.

GK: I insist on training as a prelude to workstation evaluations. Ideally, I prefer group trainings, but when this is not possible, I will spend some extra time with the person to fill them in. I am preparing a short, PowerBook presentation to do for these inevitable one-on-one evals. I find evaluations much less effective if people don't understand why I am telling them to reposition the monitor, adjust the chair, get a glare screen, lighten up on the keyboard, etc. I also am trying to get people self-managing—they should be able to adjust a workstation to their needs without having a consultant with them. My training session is a one-hour presentation with very high-quality slides. It covers:

- A basic review of the situation—some statistics, impact on people and businesses.
- Injury descriptions and anatomy—when you know how the body works, you know what can injure it.

- Ergonomics—the place to start with prevention. Principles of work-station arrangement.
- Prevention strategies—bringing good health to the machine, staying warm, relieving the eyes, managing stress, learning the software, drinking water, etc. The point is that the best ergonomics will not save you if you push the body too far, and CTD [Cumulative Trauma Disorder] prevention is a shared effort—both management and staff are responsible.

I then perform workstation evaluations in one of two modes. For those at high risk (I provide a list of criteria) I do a comprehensive eval based on a document I have designed. It takes about an hour, includes Polaroid shots and a written report. For the rest, I do a more informal eval. In either case, I make what changes I can on the spot—chair adjustment, monitor position, etc.—and recommend products as needed. My clients receive a copy of the Onsight resource guide.

I provide a limited selection of products directly. My strategy is to deal in those items I find are most commonly needed—wrist rests, Handeze Gloves, LifeGuard software, a good articulating keyboard tray, and more recently the Kensington trackballs and Thinking Mouse. My clients have the option of asking me not to provide products directly, and in any case I will point them to other sources for the many objects I do not represent.

I have just added a manager's training session to the lineup. It is also one hour. The first half is a condensed version of staff training, and the second half is specific to management, discussing:

- Importance of the supervisory relationship to safety and stress
- Time and production management
- Job design
- Micro-breaks and how they enhance productivity
- Importance of sufficient job/computer training—stress and wasted hand movement
- High-risk conditions—new hires, new technology, deadline crunches, etc.
- Watching for symptoms

My clients? Large and small. The large clients are the ones who are just beginning to understand the issue and want to start with small steps. My presence tends to help the awareness spread as people discover the comfort and benefits of safe computing, and managers discover they don't need to be afraid of the work. Sometimes I get into a larger organization through a particular workgroup who independently requested my services.

My ideal client company is five to one hundred people. Those who hire me either are witnessing problems and are concerned, or are smart enough to see the wisdom of the work, the reality of the risk. Onsight has worked with two clients on the development of a company policy statement.

TC: What is involved in a worksite evaluation?

GK: First I find out about the person—have they had symptoms? Do they wear glasses? How much time on the computer? What is the job/task description?, etc. All of the comments and adjustments I make are based on the intensity of their repetitive tasks (not just computing) and their degree of risk. If someone only sits an hour a day and computes for fifteen minutes, I'm not going to make a big deal out of their bad chair or the fact that their monitor is at an angle.

In part, here is what else I consider:

The general desk—is there enough space? Sharp edges? Need to reach shelves often? Does it have a document holder? What are the various components of their computer?

Keyboard—is it placed in front? Does it have an alternative design? Is there an adjustable tray? What is their wrist posture?

Mouse/trackball—position, type, intensity of use.

Monitor—height, brightness/contrast. Is it kept clean? Is there glare from the screen?

The computer—is it sufficient for their work? Are files easily accessed? Is their drive/network well organized? Do they need training in commonly used software?

I adjust their chair on the spot, usually the first thing we do. In almost all cases I find that people don't know how to operate all the controls (particularly back height and angle) or have never been taught how to sit. Mostly I try to give people the option of reclining, and encourage them to spend more time with their weight against the back of the chair to relieve their trunk muscles. Obviously, this means getting all other components—keyboard and monitor—in the correct relationship. When someone has the wrong chair, I make recommendations accordingly. Often I find that overweight people need special chairs, or shorter people who are unable to sit back because the seat pan is too deep on the standard-issue company chair—ergonomic though they may be.

Other issues I look at are telephone usage—I recommend lots of headset phones—as well as lighting, noise, and temperature.

A comprehensive evaluation takes about an hour, including about ten minutes of just watching someone work at the computer as I make notes in my eval form. Lately I have been using my video camera to tape people while they type and show them details of their technique to adjust, like extending the fingers or thumb, bending the wrist, leaving the hands pronated when they aren't keying, etc. Generally, they were not aware of these things and find them enlightening.

The most common problem by far is that keyboards are positioned way too high, often aggravated by wrong chairs. If someone also spends a lot of time writing or working with paper, the conflict of needing different heights for these tasks is often hard to resolve. The desk layout may not allow for a keyboard tray, or if one is used they may be forced to constantly slide it in and out from under the desk so they have space at their writing surface.

I also see many keyboard trays that I consider poorly designed. Some have no wrist support or a small, hard pad. Most are not wide enough for the mouse/trackball, forcing people to place them on the desk and reach for them, preventing them from being able to sit back in the chair.

I find people often are poorly trained in some of the most basic operations of the computer. For example, on the Macintosh you can press the tab key to move to the next entry field in a dialog box, and it being highlighted one simply needs to type and what was there will automatically be deleted. Still, many people reach for the mouse and click and drag on text, or press the delete key when it is completely unnecessary. This alone represents a tremendous amount of hand use that is avoidable.

TC: What can an employee do to maintain good relationships at work while protecting themselves from injury?

GK: The very first thing is to educate themselves. They can't win the support of a supervisor if they can't responsibly make a case for why they are experiencing discomfort, and they will not effect needed changes if they can't help the supervisor understand why the changes are needed and what they will accomplish. I have been trying to focus more on the gains in productivity that result from making people comfortable. I believe that we have an epidemic of early, unnecessary fatigue in the office in any given day. People simply don't work as well, even if they are only having slight discomfort. I also believe most people don't realize they are getting tired earlier than they should, and take their discomforts for granted as "part of the job."

Injury prevention is actually a *secondary* benefit of what is primarily good for the company in the computer-based office.

Once someone is injured, I think a supervisor simply wants to be assured that the person will be able to perform their job. When faced with the option of providing an accommodation (they may need to be told it is the law under the ADA) or else the extreme costs of having that employee on disability on top of paying temps or overtime, I think it is the wiser business decision to support that injured worker ergonomically. Even wiser—don't let the injuries happen in the first place.

TC: Gary, there are hundreds of products out there calling themselves "ergonomically-designed." What are your thoughts on the market today and what can we as consumers look for?

GK: My approach is to school people in the principles of ergonomics, not to trust anything simply because it says it's ergonomic. It has much more to do with application to a given situation or adjustability.

For instance, wrist rests. The point is to not create pressure on the wrist, so they need to be soft. Some are rounded, so, in my view, focus more pressure on a smaller area, potentially aggravating pressure in the carpal tunnel. Any wrist rest will increase pressure on the wrist if the desk is too high or the chair is too low, so for any ergonomic product, the entire work setting must be taken into account.

Chairs are probably the most heinous area of misrepresentation. I see chairs with fixed armrests that are narrow and hard being promoted as computer chairs, which for many people would place pressure on the ulnar nerve at the elbow, require muscular effort just to keep the arms on the rests, or interfere with the arms, leading them to be squeezed into the body or abducted away—all uncomfortable, all increasing the potential for fatigue and muscular strain.

More to the point, the choice of a chair has so much to do with the person's body size and weight, and the types of tasks they perform. If writing is a significant part of the work, the chair needs to be able to tilt forward with the person, or else the angle at hip is lessened and circulation to the legs decreased. The chair discussion can go on for a long time, and I feel that anyone doing extended computer/desk work should get properly advised on what chair is appropriate for them. Unfortunately I have encountered clients who simply chose one out of a catalog, or were poorly advised by an office supply salesperson who did not have sufficient knowledge of ergonomic principles.

In the case of monitors, I find that the issue is most often height, yet most monitor arms only rotate, tilt, or swing sideways. Usually monitor height is managed with the computer, phone books, or plastic trays like those from VuRyte. In the case of a shared workstation I like to see a fully adjustable monitor arm that each person who sits down can adjust to their needs.

Anything that is adjustable should be *easily* adjustable. Knobs that require pinching, or strong grip, and make someone exert a lot of force to tighten are not really in the spirit of good ergonomics if they strain the body to use them.

Articulating keyboard trays are also a bit complex. Many are not wide enough for a mouse or trackball, so cause people to have to stretch forward, doing awkward reaches and being taken away from the chair back. Many desk setups just don't have space for a tray, but at the same time have the typical problem of the table being too high for the keyboard. Often I find myself forced into compromise, often by recommending a footrest, which I prefer not to do because it limits postural options. I have seen many keyboard trays with poor or no wrist surfaces. Most people need a soft surface for the hands to rest when not typing. I've also seen trays that are difficult to move in and out from under the desk, that tear hosiery, and generally interfere with the legs. There is one particular design which has a retractable mouse tray, but it has a little lip around the edge, so that a mouse pad is unable to lie flat, making it very hard to track well with the mouse.

I see a great deal of "computer furniture" that has a little keyboard drawer which is not height-adjustable, so likely to fit few people comfortably. They also tend to promote sitting too close to the monitor since these desks are usually not very deep. This also means little room under the table to stretch the legs or achieve a variety of acceptable postures. Some of these tables also mandate that the monitor is placed at an angle to the user, promoting twisted and/or leaning postures. Definitely not ergonomic!

And, as with any product, invest in quality. Why spend money on something that will not last? If it is cheap, it is less likely to be well made, so I tend to be wary of ergonomic accessories found in the office supply stores. One exception to that is my document holder. Plastic, sticks to the side of the monitor, has a little roller that grasps the paper, four bucks. I love it.

TC: Any favorite products?

GK: I am a fan of LifeGuard reminder software. I think people really need the little breaks to breathe, close the eyes, get a drink, stand up for a second, etc. Since we lose track of time so easily at the computer, a reminder program is really valuable. I depend on it. I more often than not recommend wrist support, but take time to explain that one should rest on it in between typing, rather than rely on it during typing. Also, as I said, make sure that everything stays in good relationship—careful not to push the keyboard away from the body, or be drawn in too close to the monitor.

I am not a fan of the mouse. I feel it is very stressful to the hand, so I like to see people using trackballs if their work is cursor-intensive. It is ususaly necessary to explain the click-lock function which spares the need to ever have to do sustained pressing of the button and squeezing of the device. Still, very often for graphic artists, a trackball works poorly for drawing, so a pen pad can be good, if the extra demands it places on desk space can be accommodated. I am also a fan of the new Kensington Thinking Mouse, which, for a mouse, relieves a lot of strain to the hand by virtue of its design, and has very powerful programmability features, including click-lock, double-click with a single button, on-screen pop-up menus, etc.

I believe in keeping the hands warm, that circulation is key to safety for high repetitive use of the hands. This is particularly true of cool spaces, and of many women who tend more often to have thinner wrists, so less blood flow to the hands. Fingerless gloves like Handeze serve the purpose well.

Anyone who spends significant time on the phone should, in my view, use a headset phone. I think these will become more and more common. People just should not be cradling the phone between the ear and the shoulder. I recommend them a lot.

For more information about Onsight, or to contact Gary Karp personally:

Onsight
1510 Eddy Street, Suite 1511
San Francisco, CA 94115
(415) 749-1983

CHAPTER NINE

Exercises to Stretch and Strengthen

Exercise is an integral part of prevention and recovery from repetitive stress injuries like Carpal Tunnel Syndrome. Numerous health care practitioners I interviewed mentioned a sedentary lifestyle as a contributing factor in many cases of repetitive stress injuries. Warming up before work, cooling down at the end of a long day, stretching out stiff muscles, or strengthening with light weights to rehabilitate an injured hand are some of the ways exercise can fit into your treatment plan. Your first exercises should simply help you regain full range of motion in your hands and upper body. Strengthening comes later. For now, especially if you've just ended a period of immobilization, stretching is an excellent start.

It's important to stress that any program of exercise *must be approved by your health care professional before you start.* Exercise and stretching should feel good. If you experience an increase in symptoms, stop and consult your doctor or therapist.

The Advantages of Stretching

Regular, gentle stretching is good for your mind *and* your body; it's easy, costs nothing, and can be done nearly anywhere, anytime. Stretching improves your range of motion, relaxes muscle tension, increases circulation, and can help prevent injuries. Stretching the entire upper body at the beginning and the end of your day relieves tension and relaxes muscles.

It is much easier to injure a tight, tense muscle than a loose, relaxed one. When muscles tighten up their blood supply is diminished, as is their ability to rid themselves of metabolic waste build-up. And as most of us can attest, one tense muscle soon leads to more. At the end of the work day, our entire *bodies* ache. Stretching gently at regular intervals during the day can prevent that soreness and fatigue and leave you feeling refreshed when your day is over.

Stretching should be done slowly and easily . . . no bouncing, jerking, or painful overstretching. You should be able to breathe naturally during a stretch. Farther is *not* better! The "no pain, no gain" theory of physical fitness has no place here—none of these stretches or exercises should feel painful. When you are finished you should feel loose and warmed up, not sore. Proceed slowly. Make stretching a regular part of your daily routine, and you will notice a difference in how you feel and move.

Whole-Body Stretches

Begin your stretching routine with these easy stretches for the parts of the body those of us with repetitive strain injuries tend to ignore. Keep your *entire body* in good shape, and your hands and arms will reap the benefits.

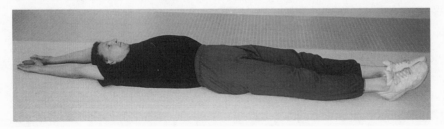

Figure 26

Lie on your back, with your arms extended over your head, fingers and toes pointed as you stretch as far as you comfortably can. The small of your back should be flat against the floor. Don't arch your back. Inhale and stretch, hold for five seconds, and relax as you exhale.

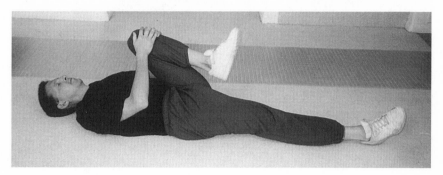

Figure 27

Next, pull your left leg toward your chest. Keep your head flat on the floor. Hold the leg for thirty seconds. Relax and repeat with the right leg.

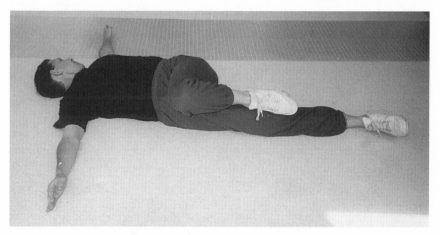

Figure 28

Still flat on the floor, stretch your arms out to the side (like a "T"). Bend your left leg up to your chest as before, then slowly bring it over the right leg. Keep your shoulders flat on the floor as much as you can, and turn your head to look toward the left arm. You should feel a stretch in your hip and lower back. Hold for thirty seconds, then relax. Repeat with the right leg.

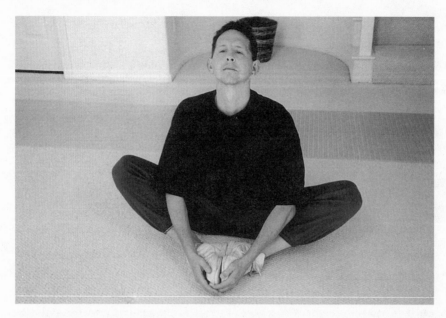

Figure 29

Sitting up now, position the soles of your feet together. Holding your feet in your hands, gently pull yourself forward from the hips. Don't round your shoulders or allow your head to flop downward. Hold for thirty seconds or so, then relax.

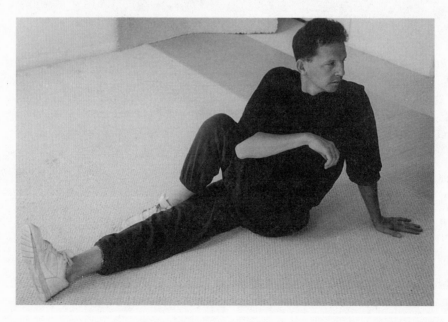

Figure 30

From your sitting position, straighten your right leg, keeping the left leg bent. Cross your left leg over the right, resting your left foot just above the outside of your right knee. Resting your left hand behind you, slowly turn to look over your left shoulder as you rotate your upper body to the left. Hold for twenty seconds, then repeat for the right side.

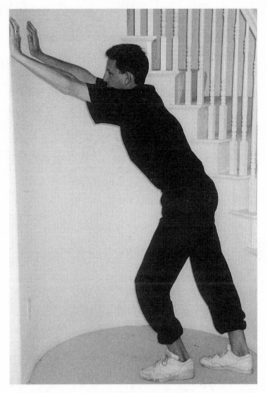

In a standing position, stand about a foot away from a wall and lean on it with your forearms. Bend your left leg, with the left foot on the ground in front of you a few inches from the wall. Keep the right leg straight. Slowly lean forward from the hips while you feel a stretch in the calf of the right leg. Hold for thirty seconds—gently, don't bounce. Repeat by bending the right leg.

Figure 31

Stretches for the Hand

Your hands are an amazing and complex combination of bones (twenty-seven in all), muscles, ligaments, and nerves, all working together to allow you to perform a nearly endless variety of tasks. Those of us who have been ordered by a concerned physician to "Stop using those hands!" can attest to the total helplessness we feel without the ability to grasp, type, write, button, pinch, or any of the other thousands of movements we used to take for granted.

Overuse can leave the muscles of the hand feeling stiff, weak, or sore. There may be a lack of grip strength (although this is generally thought to come from the forearm), or problems with coordination, especially with small, intricate tasks. Massage, moist heat, and paraffin baths are all effective in relieving some of these symptoms, but with your physician's approval you should also begin to stretch and strengthen the hand to achieve full rehabilitation.

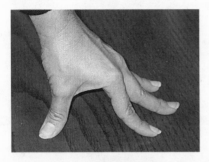

A simple stretch for the hand starts with the palm flat down on a table, fingers spread. Arch the hand by pressing down with the thumb and little finger (almost like a mini-pushup for the hand). Count to five, then release. Repeat ten to fifteen times, two or three times a day.

Figure 32

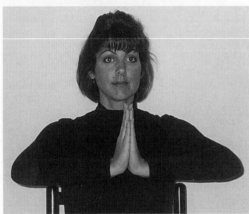

Gently flexing and extending the wrist can help you increase your range of motion as well. Place the palms of your hands together and push, raising your elbows to increase the stretch. In the beginning, five to ten seconds may be as long as you can hold this position without strain. Repeat five times.

Figure 33

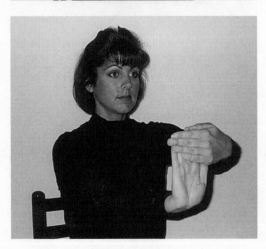

Another simple stretch involves holding the right arm out in front of you, with the elbow straight. With your left hand, grasp the fingers of the right hand and gently pull back for ten seconds. Release, and repeat with the left hand. This exercise can be reversed—grasping the right hand, pull it down so that the fingertips point toward the floor.

Figure 34

To gently mobilize the wrist and carpal bones, hold your hand straight out, thumb side up. Slowly trace a small circle in the air with your fingertips, moving only your wrist. Trace ten circles, followed by ten figure eights. Repeat with your other hand. There are many ways to vary this exercise— try it with your hand in a fist, tracing with your knuckles. Point your hand down at the floor or straight up at the ceiling. Experiment with what feels best to you.

Finally, stretch your thumb and each finger one at a time by pulling back on them gently. Give your hands a shake to get the circulation going, and finish up by just letting your hands dangle, completely limp, at your sides.

You can also stretch the fingers while relaxing in the bathtub, with the hands submerged in comfortably warm water.

Stretches for the Arms and Shoulders

The following stretches, with the exception of the Doorway Stretch, can be performed right at your desk, and I recommend them before, during, and after the work day. We hold a lot of tension in this upper-body area, especially the shoulders.

Arm Stretch
Lace your fingers together above your head, palms facing up. Stretch your arms up and slightly back.

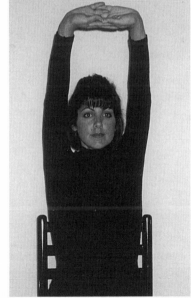

Figure 35

Shoulder Shrug

Slowly shrug the shoulders as high as you can, hold for a count of five, then release. Repeat five times.

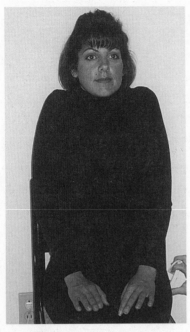 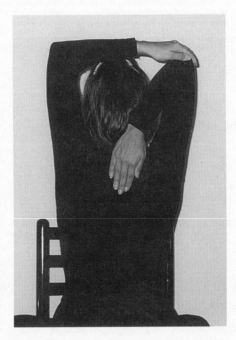

Figure 36   Figure 37

Shoulder Stretch

Bring the right hand behind your head to the upper back. Gently pull the right elbow back and downward with the left hand, moving the right hand down toward the center of the upper back. Repeat on opposite side.

Shoulder Rotation

Clasp hands behind the back. With arms extended straight, slowly lift arms upward.

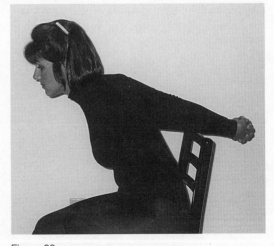

Figure 38

Doorway Stretch

Stand in a doorway, with the left arm raised up to shoulder level. Bend the elbow, with the fingers relaxed and pointing upward. Align the front of the shoulder with the doorjamb [see photo], arm resting against the wall. Stretch forward. Experiment with changing the angle of your arm and feel how this changes the muscles being stretched. Switch arms.

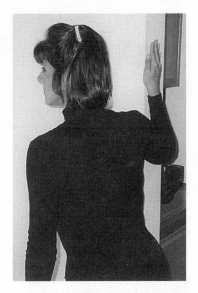

Figure 39

Stretches for the Neck

Your neck muscles are some of the hardest-working muscles in your entire body. Those muscles help you not only move your head and neck, but also chew, swallow, and talk—not to mention holding the approximately ten-pound weight of your head upright! It's important to be aware of the neck's involvement in the development of overuse injuries. The neck must be kept as mobile and flexible as possible to ensure that there is little or no pressure on the nerve roots coming out of the cervical spine. Reducing muscle tension and pressure in the neck optimizes the functioning of the nerves going down into the arm.

Simple mobility exercises are necessary to keep the neck flexible. These exercises should be done as often as possible, at least three times a day. I recommend one of the sessions each day be performed while standing under a comfortably hot shower.

Figure 40—Sit or stand in a normal position with the head facing straight ahead.

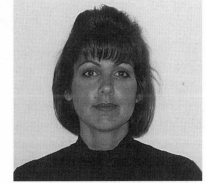

Figure 40

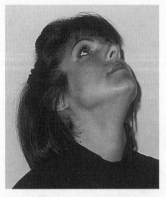

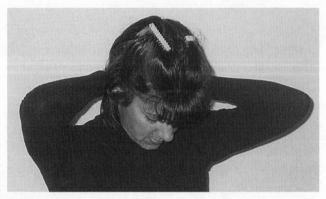

Figure 41   Figure 42

Figure 41—Tilt the head back as far as is comfortable. This should be a *smooth* backward motion—not done in a jerking manner. Do this three times. Do not force the neck back—just let it drop back naturally enough to feel a stretch along the muscles in the front of your neck.

Figure 42—Lacing your fingers behind your head, gently pull the head forward, touching the chin to the chest. Repeat three times. Return to a normal position of looking straight ahead.

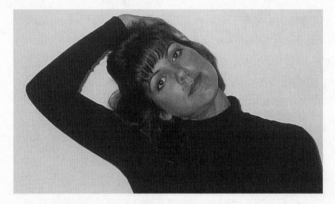

Figure 43

Figure 43—While facing forward, place the right hand over the head to the left ear. Gently pull the head to the right so that the right ear touches the right shoulder. This is done three times. Keep looking forward and do not rotate the head, but instead laterally flex the head as much and as painlessly as possible. Do the same with the left side.

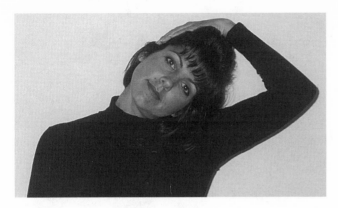

Figure 44

Place the right hand on the back of your head, pulling your head forward and to the right. Repeat three times, then do the left side.

Figure 44—Roll the head around counter-clockwise, three times, smoothly and without jerking motions, in as wide a range of motion as is painlessly possible.

Last of all, roll the head around clockwise as described above.

These exercises should feel comfortable. Again, do *not* attempt any exercise if pain is present before, during, or after you've finished. Care should be taken to stretch only within a comfortable range.

Stretches for the Chest and Upper Back

Don't overlook the chest and upper back when going through your stretching routine. Stretching the chest and upper back will help you to relax and breathe deeply, as well as keep your spine in alignment and your posture nice and straight.

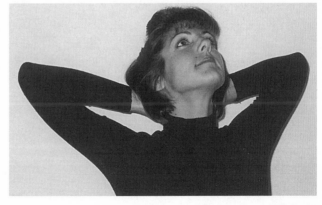

Chest Stretch—Figure 45
Lace your fingers behind your head. Stretch back, imagining that you are trying to make your elbows touch.

Figure 45

Upper Back Stretch #1—Figure 46

Place the left hand on the right shoulder. Hold the left arm above the elbow with the right hand. Slowly pull the left elbow, stretching toward the right shoulder. Repeat for the opposite side.

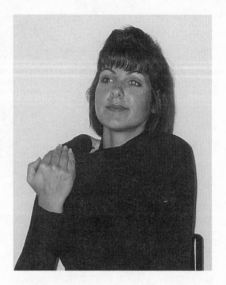

Figure 46

Upper Back Stretch #2—Figure 47

In a standing position, place both hands out in front of you, braced against a wall, file cabinet, ledge, etc., shoulder-width apart. Feet should be slightly apart, with hips positioned directly above your feet. Knees are slightly bent. Let your upper body drop down and forward, stretching out your upper back. You can adjust the position of your arms or the degree of bend in your knees to stretch different muscles. Hold for at least thirty seconds.

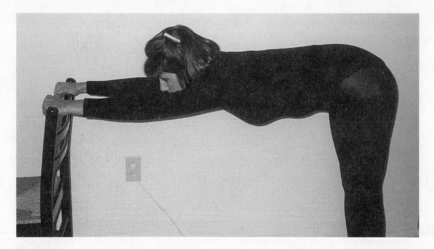

Figure 47

Full Back Stretch—Figure 48

Bend forward as far as you can, dropping the head, shoulders, and arms forward.

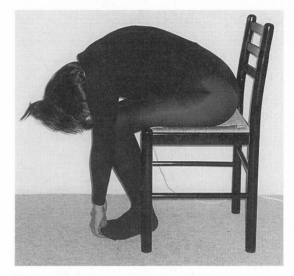

Figure 48

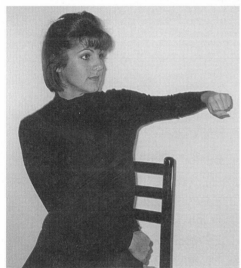

Figure 49

Upper Body Rotation—Figure 49

Grasp the left hip with the right hand. Bend the left arm and raise to shoulder height. Rotate the upper body to the left while pulling on the hip with the right hand. Repeat for opposite side.

Side Rotation—Figure 50

Place the left hand on the hip (be careful not to hyperextend the wrist). With the right arm extended overhead, slowly stretch the upper body to the left. Repeat for opposite side.

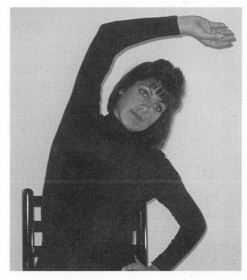

Figure 50

Strengthening Exercises

Once initial inflammation subsides and your physician approves a program of rehabilitative exercise, it is time to begin to build up the muscles in the arms and upper body to allow them to function as fully as possible and to divert pressure off the vulnerable areas of the wrist. *These exercises are not recommended during periods of pain or numbness,* but rather before symptoms develop or after they resolve.

Arm-strengthening exercises should only be done when there is no pain or inflammation present when examining your elbow and forearm. If you feel discomfort in the arms, place a forearm brace on the arm *below* where it hurts, and apply ice to the injured part of the elbow on a daily basis until the inflammation subsides. If any pain is felt during or after the exercises, talk with your health care practitioner before trying again.

A program with weights, exercise bands, and/or isometrics, approved by your health care practitioner, can help you not only to recover but to increase your strength and muscle tone, preventing any further problems from occurring.

Strengthening Exercises For The Hands

Some CTS patients have obtained good results from exercising the hand using a special kind of therapy putty. Even gripping a rubber ball hard for a few seconds will help to improve strength and flexibility. Also widely available are hand exercisers made of hard plastic grips and a thick spring; I personally don't care for the rigid plastic and find it provides too much resistance for an injured hand. Stick with the softer exercisers for an easier workout. I use the Rhino Gripper™ [see Therapy Skill Builders in Appendix C], an inexpensive foam device contoured for the hand which can be used in numerous ways to tone and strengthen key muscle groups in the hands and forearms.

Strengthening Exercises for the Wrists

When you are ready to begin strengthening the wrist muscles, add light weights to your routine. You can use a light dumbbell (start with just a pound

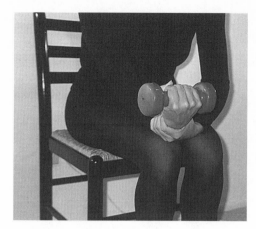

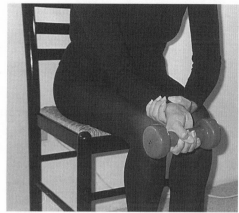

Figure 51   Figure 52

or two and build up slowly) and if you have access to an exercise bench, great. Look around your home or office and make the most of what you find to set up a place to exercise—a coffee table, ironing board, soup cans instead of weights—use your imagination!

Wrist curls are performed like this: using an exercise bench or other support for your forearm, hold the dumbbell in your right hand with your wrist extending out past the bench. With your palm facing up, flex your wrist and bring the dumbbell up no more than one to two inches. Repeat ten times, then switch to the left arm. Next, repeat the exercise twice more with the arm in the following positions: palm down, again raising the weight no more than one to two inches, and palm in, with the thumb up, working the wrist back and forth.

Strengthening Exercises for the Forearms

Put your arm up in front of you, grasp the arm just above the elbow with the other hand, then make and release a fist. You should be able to feel and even see the forearm muscles at work. The muscles that control the hand strength are in the forearm, not in the wrist, and this area is frequently overlooked as a source of potential irritation.

Curls with light weights (no more than three to five pounds each to start) can build up strength in the forearms. This exercise can be performed

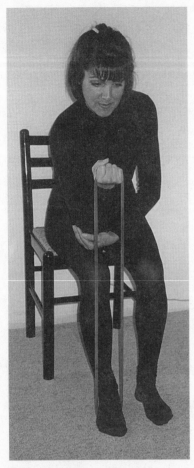

Figure 53

sitting or standing: hold a dumbbell in each hand, arms at your sides and palms facing backward. Bring the arms up, and in one continuous movement, turn the arms so that palms end up facing the ceiling. Reverse the movement and return the arms to starting position, palms again facing backward.

Strengthening Exercises for the Biceps

Conditioning of the biceps can be accomplished with weights or the use of an elastic exercise band. Variations on this exercise involve a simple change in palm orientation—try five repetitions each with the palm facing up, facing down, then with palms facing each other. Remember to keep your wrists absolutely straight during this exercise.

Exercise bands or tubing can be very beneficial in strengthening the arms and upper back. They come in a variety of lengths and thicknesses. In Figure 53 Kristie is demonstrating a simple bicep curl.

Strengthening Exercises for the Neck

Here are a few simple isometric exercises to improve neck strength:

Figure 54—Sit comfortably in a chair, feet flat on the floor and back straight. Place your right hand against the right side of your head, and press your head against the resistance of your hand. Repeat on the left.

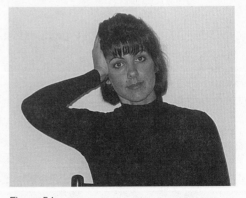

Figure 54

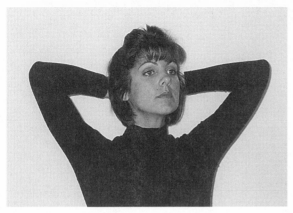

Figure 55

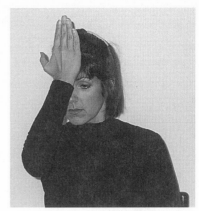

Figure 56

Figure 55—Next, lace your fingers behind your head. Push your head backward while resisting with your hands.

Figure 56—Finally, place one palm against your forehead. Press forward while *resisting* with your hand. Hold each press for five to ten seconds, and repeat five times in the beginning, working up to ten repetitions each.

Strengthening the Upper Back

To strengthen the muscles of the upper back, loop exercise tubing to a doorknob or other stationary object. Hold the band with both hands, elbows between waist and shoulder level, and pull the band back, as in Figure 57. Feel your shoulders pull back and your shoulder blades draw together. Repeat five times, then raise your elbows to shoulder height. As you repeat the exercise, feel the difference that changing the elbow position has on the muscles you are working.

DO NOT CONTINUE ANY MOVEMENT THAT FEELS PAINFUL.

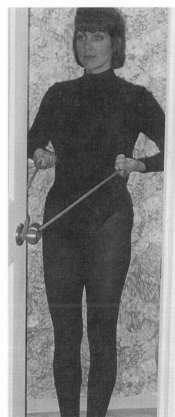

Figure 57

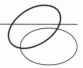

Living with Carpal Tunnel Syndrome and Repetitive Strain Injuries: *Your Stories*

One of the things I found most helpful as a patient was simply listening to the stories of other people like me. They gave me factual information, suggestions for self-help, support, and more important, let me know that I wasn't the only person struggling to get my coat unzipped! For this book, I sent out questionnaires through the mail, distributed surveys through doctors' offices, posted innumerable messages throughout the Internet, and made hundreds of telephone calls. You responded with hundreds of personal stories. I was touched not only by your experiences but by your willingness to share information in the hope that it might help just one other person.

Certain themes ran throughout these stories: frustration in finding a doctor who cared, a treatment that worked or even a correct diagnosis, pressure at work to perform at a level no longer physically possible, anger at the Workers' Compensation system, weariness from living with chronic pain and physical limitations. However, there was also ingenuity—the suggestions for ways to adapt the environment were wonderfully creative—and there was hope that by sharing information about doctors and products and treatment we could not only feel better but ideally prevent someone else from going through what we did.

I couldn't possibly print them all, but here are some of the thoughts, experiences, and suggestions you shared with me. Where I was asked, I've protected the identity of the contributor. At the risk of being redundant, use your common sense and, if appropriate, obtain the advice of your own health care professional if you'd like to try any of the suggestions below.

Robin Coutellier

My diagnosis is tendinitis affecting the ulnar tendon (which goes through a narrow point known as "Guyon's canal," similar to the carpal tunnel). The chronic inflammation led to a subsequent diagnosis of Carpal Tunnel Syndrome. I had a third problem of a compressed nerve affecting the carpal ulnaris flexor tendon (baby finger). I had surgery on my left wrist and elbow on 11/25/91. The wrist surgery was a carpal tunnel release and a "Guyon's canal" release. The elbow surgery was a cubital tunnel release, which freed the compressed nerve that was impairing the use of my baby finger. I had a local anesthetic and was awake (although sedated) during the surgery. I was sent home the same day as soon as I felt up to making the trip. I have a sensitivity to narcotic pain relievers such as codeine, so I was only able to take ibuprofen for the pain. The ibuprofen was very effective, although I did take about 800 mg. every three hours, including in the middle of the night, being very careful to eat something first. Until the "soft cast" was removed a week later, I needed someone to cook for me and help me bathe, but I was able to dress myself (very loose clothing). I rested my arm and wrists on a large pillow almost continuously, keeping them above heart level whenever possible, on the doctor's advice. My right wrist improved amazingly during the ten weeks I was off work. I went back to work half days for a month, then increased to five hours per day. My right hand became increasingly more painful to use and was soon back to where it was before my disability leave. So much for a long rest! I very gradually built back up to eight hours a day. My first eight-hour day was 12/24/92, a year after the surgery.

I still experience pain in my left wrist and hands, although it's not usually as sharp as it was before the surgery. I haven't progressed as well as other people who have had surgery, partly because I've returned to the same type of work, although it's much more varied and "adjusted" than when I was first injured. I'm not satisfied enough with the surgery on my left wrist to have it done on the right one yet. The doctor says he doesn't consider a patient stable until two years after surgery.

Along these lines, I spoke with a woman who had had the same problem, and it took five surgeries (three on one, two on the other) over a period of five years to recover. That sounds like a life sentence to someone who is just now beginning to feel the effects of RSI, but after two and a half years, it sounds more to me like there might be some light at the end of the tunnel.

Some of the things I've done to help me cope and get things done since I've been injured are:

• Most books, even paperbacks, have been too heavy to hold or too hard to hold open for very long. What I do now is break the book into sections of 50–100 pages each, then use a large "chip-clip" to hold it open. I have to be careful not to use too much pressure when squeezing the clip open, sometimes using the weight of my hand rather than my fingers to squeeze it open.

• I saw a mechanical scrubber on a late-night infomercial and ordered it (about $100). It's lightweight and cleans, polishes, etc., just about anything, with a lot of attachments, even one to clean computer keyboards. I ordered it but have not really put it to use yet, in part because removing the attachments is difficult and, in the case of the bottle brush, nearly impossible.

• I bought a very lightweight (~8 lbs.) vacuum cleaner by Panasonic with easy-to-use attachments (though I do find the attachments hard to remove!). It's not self-propelled (which would make the vacuum heavier), but it pulls itself forward and back with only minor effort from me. It's called the Panasonic Jet-Flo, and the model number is MC-5107. It costs about $200.

• I use plastic utensils and paper plates, bowls, and cups, and a lightweight "camping" mug for hot drinks. They're much easier to deal with not only by weight, but since I throw them away, there are few, if any, dishes to wash (though I've discovered that washing dishes, if done in moderation, actually makes the wrists feel better, getting the circulation going and improving the range of motion). These items can be bought in bulk for a very low price.

• I've been making good use of the salad bars at Safeway and other supermarkets. The veggies are usually very fresh, and I don't have to chop anything. The salad bars are also good for obtaining pre-cut stir-fry ingredients.

• I finally convinced my landlord to allow me to have a garage door opener installed (at my expense).

• I have a shoemaker put Velcro on my shoes (at a cost of $10-$15) so I don't have to tie the laces; this is imperative if you're going to have hand/wrist surgery. Also, if you're going to have surgery, get some pull-on pants with an elastic waist so you don't have to deal with a zipper.

[Author's note: From personal experience, also be sure you choose shirts with sleeves loose enough to pass your bulky cast through. I ended up having to cut the sleeves on three shirts in order to make an opening wide enough.]

• I was unable to drive for six weeks after my surgery and took the bus everywhere. I was able to buy a "disabled/senior" monthly bus pass for $5, as opposed to about $30-$35 for the normal adult monthly bus pass. I bought them at Lucky via the normal checkout counter.

• Most physical therapists will have someone with an RSI start exercising with small weights (1/2, 1, 2 lbs.). At sporting goods stores, these can be somewhat expensive. I've bought fishing weights at Payless for 39 cents to $1, depending on the weight. Not only is it extremely cheap, but you can get very precise that way, buying by the ounce, i.e., 4 oz., 6 oz., 8 oz., etc., along with 1- or 2-lb weights (adding only 4, 6, or 8 oz. at a time between pounds can make the transition much easier and is less likely to put too much strain on the joints).

• Using a very lightweight blow dryer—or getting a perm—is much easier on the hands/wrists.

• Hot and cold contrast baths are very good for increasing circulation. My hand therapist advised me to always do this just before exercising. If you have a dual sink, fill one side with warm-hot water, and the other with cold water. Use dishpans or other containers if you have a single sink. Start out putting hand(s) in warm water for one minute, then switch to cold for one minute, etc. for ten minutes, ending on the cold cycle. Move hands gently in the warm water, but keep them relatively still in the cold water. I have a book on the windowsill in front of me and read, which is a great distraction. I use my nearby microwave with three-stage cooking (a beep a minute for three minutes) to tell me when each minute is up. Sometimes I put baby oil in the water.

Dan Wallach ("The Typing Injury FAQ Archive")

It all began simply enough. I was Joe-random Berkeley undergrad who landed a summer internship in 1991. Everything that could have gone wrong, did. They gave me terrible furniture—the keyboard was too high, the chair wasn't adjustable, and the keyboard was mushy and annoying. Still, I was obsessive about working, not taking breaks, etc. Combine that with one-hour drives from Berkeley to Mountain View and back again, so I could see friends. Stir in the home video game machines my roommate just got (I was the consummate video game junkie). Oh yeah, I also played racquetball. Duh. This is as much a recipe for disaster as you could imagine. Sure enough, I woke up one morning after video gaming the night before with my right hand tingling like mad. I asked around and some friends who'd suffered with this before pointed me to a medical center in San Jose who really knew their stuff, except they had a two-week backlog! My employer initially sent me to a local drive-up clinic which prescribed me ibuprofen horse-pills (which only upset my stomach) and a splint (which didn't fit).

At the time, wacky keyboards were only something people had "heard of" but never seen. My employers were very nice—if I could find it, they'd buy it for me. So, I started looking, and I eventually compiled a list of some vendors, based on what I heard from folks on the Internet.

The medical center in San Jose diagnosed me with tendinitis. They made me custom wrist-splints, which saved me. They also prescribed icing, exercises, and other stuff which never seemed to have a terribly great effect. They only attacked my physical symptoms and never evaluated my work environment or life in general. So, I'd do something boneheaded and set myself back a week or two and have to climb back up again. This lasted the whole summer, then I went back to Berkeley. This had the greatest effect on me. Suddenly, I wasn't working eight to ten hour days in front of the computer. Instead, I planned my time better and spent maybe half that time for a semester. I felt like an idiot walking around with wrist splints, although people were very nice to me. I discovered that driving my great little sports car puts me in great pain—one hour of driving is worse than hours and hours of typing, wrist braces or no. Needless to say, I started re-evaluating each and every aspect of my life. By this time, I was reposting my list of keyboards to the Internet as the Typing Injury FAQ. I also collected every online document I could find into my ftp archive.

By the time the next summer rolled around, I went back to work. Despite taking great care with keyboard trays and borrowing a "good" chair, my wrists started degenerating, and I had to use the wrist braces more and more. I managed to get my new advisor at Berkeley (I was working in his research group) to shell out half the $700 cost of a Kinesis keyboard. Several of the students who also worked for my advisor and I ganged up on him and made him buy us some new chairs, too. It's just amazing how much better a new adjustable chair is compared to the old 1950s clunkers we had originally.

Life is improving now. By late 1993 I could work in comfort. I couldn't believe how much better it was than the usual crappy setup which most undergrads used. I was also paying attention to myself. If something hurt, I stopped. It sounds dumb, but it's amazing how many people keep doing what hurts them, because it doesn't hurt "much." They'll learn.

It's now 1995—over three years after my original injury. I occasionally have a relapse (like, the time I slipped on an icy street and landed on my hand—yow!), but I'm generally fine. I'm less obsessive about my work, taking more breaks and such. I also now have a height-adjustable desk and chair. I had to remove the arm-rests from the chair, but it's as comfortable as any environment I've ever experienced.

I guess I'm a success story, if there is such a thing. What did I do right? I've always been willing to "hack" my environment to fit me. At my current desk, that meant hacking my chair (funny thing—after I did it, several other people got the idea and did it too). At my last two summer jobs, it means installing a $20 Rubbermaid keyboard tray in my office desk.

Running the Typing Injury FAQ began as a favor to everybody who originally helped me find stuff on the Internet. Of course, it's almost just as easy to send your list of vendors to two people as one. And, it's also just as easy to send it to hundreds or thousands. So, I did, and it has turned out to be a rewarding hobby. I've never made any money off it, but it seems like a fairly constructive way to spend about a day a month. Of course, I'm always looking for volunteers who want to help out. There's always plenty of work to be done that neither I nor my other co-conspirators have the time for. If anybody reading this wants to donate some of their time, they can send me e-mail: dwallach@cs.princeton.edu

Dave M.

My experience started out as tendinitis on the back of both hands in May of 1992. I was typing an average of six to eight hours per day, but with frequent breaks. My company doctor pointed out that I did not have CTS (but the current condition could lead to it) and prescribed ibuprofen. Then in September of 1992, in the middle of editing a 500-page document, both hands simultaneously had shooting pains go right up through the middle fingers. I was shocked. I first consulted an acupuncturist, who treated me three or four times with no success. Then I went to a chiropractor, whose treatments seemed better at first, but when I began developing sciatic pain I stopped that. I followed that with three months of contrast baths and anti-inflammatories while under the care of an orthopedic surgeon. Finally we tried a cortisone shot. It didn't help at all. After an EMG and a nerve conduction study indicated CTS in both hands, I had a carpal tunnel ligament release on one hand to see if that would work. After a short respite (due mostly to the post-op rest), it all came back just as bad. Since then I've seen another orthopod, another acupuncturist, a physical therapist and am now seeing a myotherapist (which seems to be helping a little).

Richard W.

I'm 45 now and had carpal tunnel surgery on my left hand in November '92 and on the right in December '92. I don't know how I got this thing, but my pain began in the summer of '92 when I worked as a framing carpenter. At first it was just stiffness and tiredness that would go away when I got warmed up in the morning. Later the tingling started and would wake me up at night—I couldn't sleep more than an hour at a time, which was a real problem for me. Electrical nerve conduction tests showed blockage in the carpal tunnel and thus the surgeries in the fall and winter. Now the pain is much, much less, but a constant presence throughout the day and night. Oh, yes, most important, I don't wake up in the night anymore.

Name Withheld

I was a technical writer for ten years and typed at least eight hours a day, seventy words per minute. I never had any hand pain until I began working simultaneously on two computers. There's no way to have two computers on one desk in an ergonomically correct position, and I was constantly leaning way over to grab a mouse or type on one machine while reading text on the other. When my hands started hurting, I didn't wait to see a doctor. The first doctor I saw (a GP) wanted me to go back to my office and file a Workmen's Comp claim, then return to him so he could process me under a different account (under which he presumably receives a larger payment than my insurance would pay him). I didn't want to file a claim, and he finally gave me wrist splints and non-steroidals. These didn't help. I asked a doctor I trusted for a reference to a good neurologist. The neurologist did nerve conduction studies, determined that I was in the very early stages of carpal tunnel and had some elbow nerve damage, and gave me cortisone/Novocain injections in my wrist. The injections stopped the pain completely. However, I find that the pain returns if I work without my wrist splints or if I don't pay attention to my posture/typing position. I've made a number of changes in my work and personal habits. I don't consider myself handicapped, but I'm very protective of my hands now. Before my hands hurt, I knew that my bad work habits could cause carpal tunnel, but I figured that once I started feeling pain I would correct my habits then. I know now that once you start feeling any pain, the damage is done and it's too late. I'm just glad I caught the problem and searched for help as early as I did. One more note: every time I'm out in public wearing my wrist braces, someone asks me if I have carpal tunnel and then they tell me that they have it or one of their co-workers has it. They are eager, and sometimes desperate, to know if I've found the CURE, or at least a way to lessen the pain. Carpal Tunnel seems to be everywhere.

Name Withheld

I can commiserate with your readers. When my wrists first started hurting, I kind of knew I was in for it. The doctor I saw confirmed a repetitive stress injury and showed me some exercises. He told me to get some balance in my life and prescribed an anti-inflammatory medication. The problem with getting balance in my life is that everything I want to do involves computers. I work as a magazine editor, typing e-mail and writing news stories all day. I am also a fiction writer. I've had to sacrifice the most fulfilling part of my life, writing short stories at night, to save my hands for the work I'm paid for. If I avoid my home computer all weekend, Monday and part of Tuesday can be fairly productive. I don't yet have enough money to buy speech recognition for my home computer, which would be the best solution, so I am just trying to wait this phase out while guarding my dreams.

Name Withheld

Mine began when I came home from the hospital with a new baby. Breast feeding, pushing a cheap umbrella stroller over brick sidewalks (and lifting it downstairs), scrubbing out baby-generated stains, and not sleeping enough added up to wrist, neck, and elbow problems which worsened when I returned to computer use at work after maternity leave. I used splints at night, anti-inflammatories as needed. Four years later, I'm much better. The kid walks. The stroller was retired ages ago. Life is good.

J.S.

After three years of heavy computer work, I started feeling pain in my upper forearm near the elbow. It felt like a pulled muscle, and I ignored it for two weeks, thinking it would go away. After two weeks, the pain got worse and travelled down my forearm to my wrist. I saw a doctor right away. He referred me to a physiatrist, who did an EMG to test for Carpal Tunnel Syndrome. The EMG was negative, and the physiatrist diagnosed repetitive strain injury. I immediately notified my supervisor. A claim was issued to Workers' Compensation and I was assigned a case number. My condition got worse. I attended physical therapy, took anti-inflammatories and wore a wrist splint. Nothing fixed the problem, and I became depressed. I visited a few neurologists, more tests were done (including a spinal x-ray, an MRI, and a bone scan), and I was put on more medication. Eventually surgery was recommended, although all EMG tests were negative. I had the surgery on July 1, 1993. It was a total failure. Although the doctor performed the operation properly, I actually got worse because the scar tissue restricted my movement further. In the fall I decided to see the best doctors I could, and a top orthopedic surgeon finally gave me what I think is a proper diagnosis: tendinitis in the fingers, hand and wrist, intrinsic stiffness, and radial nerve compression. He gave me two injections of cortisone for the tendinitis and said there wasn't much more he could do while I was still beating myself up on the keyboard. Beginning in 1994, I began to take matters into my own hands. I tried to figure out how to type with the least strain on my body, and by keeping my wrist in a straight position it felt better. At work, I have been shown no support. Workers' Compensation is also a problem. I've been fighting them all the time, which doesn't help me physically. For now I'm trying to get by without therapy or medication.

James Wilson

I've been through it [surgery] twice, so I figure I can speak from a high level of experience. I'm darned glad I did it, haven't had any problems since. It had gotten so bad I'd forget I was smoking a cigarette (because I couldn't feel it between my fingers), and put my hand in my lap and burn my pants. Burned three suits like that. My right thumb was beginning to tremor, too. Plus all the nighttime discomfort. I could have delayed the surgery on the left hand; it wasn't too bad. But my insurance carrier was preparing to quit paying 100% of outpatient surgeries, and when I explained that to the doc, he said "Let's go for it!" Four grand per hand, including surgeon, anesthetist and facility. My best advice is to find a doctor who uses arthroscopic surgery.

Name Withheld

I am a grocery checker and work on a checkstand using both arms and hands. I stand, working four- to six-hour shifts, using my shoulders, arms, hands and wrists, and it all affects my back and my neck. My symptoms are pain and stiffness, and I drop things a lot. I saw one chiropractor who wasn't very helpful, then saw a local chiropractor on TV who specializes in Carpal Tunnel Syndrome. This treatment has helped very much, and my insurance covers up to a certain amount for office visits.

M.F.

My hobby is geneology, and I spend two to three hours at a time at the keyboard. I use a wrist rest to keep my wrists in a "natural" position, but my wrist is flexed while using the mouse. My right wrist burns and is painful after using the mouse for even an hour. After consulting with a neurologist and a surgeon, I was diagnosed with CTS in the right wrist and was developing it in the left. Surgery on my right wrist helped relieve the numbness and intense pain, but I continue to have some pain and weakness in the right wrist. I am also currently being treated for rheumatoid arthritis and fibromyalgia.

Eva W.

It has been a significant mental struggle and process of adaptation for me to deal with things like the changes in my work productivity and need to slow down, the need to be more dependent on other people and ask for help without feeling guilty. It would be helpful to reinforce people's ability to ask for help. "Could you please fill this in for me? I have Carpal Tunnel Syndrome and am under doctor's orders not to use my hands." As straightforward as this may sound, it took a long time for me to get up the courage to say anything. I still don't know how to respond to people who say "But your hands don't look any different." Or "Oh, RSI, the Yuppie disease." One needs to accept the reality that *real* rest and a wide margin of conservative behavior are needed. I suspect that the self-imposed need to push my limits has probably been the single most important factor that keeps me from resting and therefore hinders my recovery.

Debra S.

I work as a part-time cake decorator, and I have been diagnosed with CTS by both an M.D. and a chiropractor. The M.D. recommended that I have surgery, but I refused. I've heard bad things about the surgery and didn't want poor results. I tried splints but they weakened my wrists, and I use them only when I am doing heavy work. The treatment that helps is chiropractic—treatments to my spine and wrist provide relief for six to eight weeks. The spinal manipulations aren't permanent relief but they are very effective in controlling the pain and numbness. I also take short breaks for range of motion exercises and find swimming relieves stress and keeps my whole arm and shoulder loosened up.

Thomas B.

I've been a pipe insulator for twenty-seven years, and use a heavy staple gun to hold the insulation on the pipes and ducts. In a normal day I may pull on the staple gun 500 to 800 times. I've seen many doctors, including a G.P., an orthopedic surgeon, and a hand specialist. I had an EMG and examinations which showed bi-lateral Carpal Tunnel Syndrome and "trigger finger" in six fingers. So far I've had surgery for CTS three times (twice on the left and once on the right) and six surgical procedures to release the trigger fingers. The CTS surgeries worked, but I still have problems in my hands from the trigger finger condition. My doctor tells me I'll need at least one more surgery on each hand.

Morris D.

I am the Operations Manager for a data processing company, and work at a computer almost eight hours each day. In 1990 I began to notice numbness in my hand. I attributed this to advancing middle age (I am 43 now) and poor circulation (I have been a smoker since I was 16). The condition worsened and my hand started to go numb almost all the time. My G.P. advised me that I probably had Carpal Tunnel Syndrome and advised me to contact my Workers' Compensation Department for referral to a specialist. A neurologist diagnosed me with a "classic" case of CTS, and informed me that while many physicians used splints and cortisone to treat this, my CTS was at a stage that would only improve through surgery. My Workers' Compensation Representative told me that there were a few doctors who did laser surgery for CTS, and that the procedure was much less painful with shorter recovery time. I made an appointment with a doctor here in Atlanta, one of the first to learn this technique. This doctor was very detailed in his explanation to me about the procedure and I understood completely the risks and hopeful benefits. In May of 1994 he performed the procedure. I returned to work the following Wednesday and with the exception of slight soreness initially and a temporary loss of strength I have had absolutely no problems with the procedure, and my hand no longer goes numb.

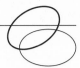

Glossary

acupuncture: A technique for treating a wide variety of conditions, acupuncture involves the insertion of very fine needles into specific points on the body. It is believed that acupuncture restores the balance of *ch'i*—the energy that makes up each being's life force.

-algia: A suffix meaning pain.

applied kinesiology: A method of muscle testing, applied kinesiology measures neurological functioning throughout the body.

arthroscope: A tool used to examine the inside of a joint, consisting of a tube and an optical device.

atrophy: Wasting away or decreasing in size; in this case, of muscle tissue.

carpal tunnel: A narrow canal in the wrist, containing tendons and the median nerve, and made up of the eight carpal bones on three sides, while the fourth is formed by the transverse carpal ligament.

Carpal Tunnel Syndrome: Inflammation and swelling around the tendons and nerve of the wrist, leading to a variety of sensory and motor symptoms including pain, numbness, and loss of strength.

cervical: Referring to the neck, i.e., the *cervical* spine.

chiropractic: A system of health care based on the premise that many musculoskeletal problems can be caused by different types of pressure on the nervous system, and that the loss of normal nerve activity can lead to disorders of certain organic systems.

computerized axial tomography: A diagnostic test providing three-dimensional, cross-sectional images of various parts of the body, using x-rays but providing far more detail than standard x-rays can. also known as **CAT scan.**

cortisone: A hormone produced naturally by the adrenal glands, cortisone may be produce synthetically and used as an anti-inflammatory agent.

cumulative trauma disorder: see **repetitive strain injury**

disk, intervertebral: Disks made of a gelatinous cartilage which separate and cushion the **vertebrae** (see below) during movement, absorb the shock caused by walking, running and jumping, permit the spinal column to bend and twist, and prevent damage to the spinal nerves.

double crush phenomenon: A regular finding among patients diagnosed with CTS, where there are two areas of nerve irritation occurring along the course of the nerve.

edema: Local or generalized swelling, caused by excess fluids in the body tissues. Edema may be caused by a number of factors, including inflammation, excess sodium retention, reduction in kidney function, or heart failure.

electromyography: The process of analyzing the electrical activity in a muscle at rest, upon insertion of a small needle, and during contraction. Also known as **EMG.**

endorphins: Chemicals produced by the brain that produce relief from pain.

ergonomics: As it relates to work-related injuries, ergonomics is the idea of creating a work environment that promotes physical health and comfort while optimizing job performance.

extension: In reference to the wrist, bending the hand back. In general, to increase the angle between any bones forming a joint. See also **hyper-.**

fascia: The fibrous membrane which separates and covers muscles, as well as connecting the skin with underlying tissues.

Fibromyalgia Syndrome: A condition involving chronic stiffness and widespread pain in the muscles, ligaments, and tendons, along with headaches, fatigue, and non-restorative sleep.

flexion: In reference to the wrist, bending the hand forward. The opposite of extension. Decreasing the angle between any bones forming a joint. See also **hyper-**.

homeopathy: A system of health care founded in the late 18th century, in which a correct remedy is one which produces reactions similar to those the patient is experiencing, activating and strengthening the patient's own system in response to the remedy.

hyper-: excessive, or beyond.

inflammation: The body's reaction to any type of injury. Signs of inflammation include redness, swelling, and pain.

interferential current therapy: Therapeutic tool using medium-frequency current to penetrate deep into joints or muscles, to increase circulation, reduce swelling and inflammation, stimulate the release of pain-reducing hormones in the body, and increase overall muscle tone.

-itis: Suffix meaning **inflammation.**

magnetic resonance imaging: A diagnostic tool which uses principles of magnetism to view tissues and organs. Also known as **MRI.**

median nerve: The median nerve starts in the neck from the area of the seventh and eighth vertebrae, and runs all the way down to the hand, carrying signals between the hand and the brain.

myo-, myos-: Prefix meaning muscle.

nerve conduction studies: Diagnostic test involving tapplying an electric stimulus to the nerve to measure the nerve's response.

neurologists: Medical doctors trained in the diagnosis and treatment of disorders of the nervous system.

occupational neuritis: see **repetitive strain injury.**

orthopedists, orthopedic surgeons: These physicians deal with many conditions of the bones, muscles, ligaments, and tendons, including Carpal Tunnel Syndrome. In cases where an injury does not respond to conservative care, the patient may be referred to a physician in this specialty to determine whether surgical intervention is needed.

osteopathy: A school of medicine which supports the theory that achieving a structural balance will bring about healing. Osteopathic physicians use the professional designation, D.O., and use a combination of manipulation and standard medicinal and surgical methods to restore health.

physiatrists: Licensed M.D.s specializing in physical medicine and rehabilitation, physiatrists treat a wide variety of acute and chronic musculoskeletal disorders.

physical therapy: Rehabilitation and restoration of normal bodily function after illness or injury through the use of patient education, therapeutic exercises, hydrotherapy, and the application of various forms of energy—electrotherapy, ultrasound, and interferential current therapy.

pronation: Referring to the hand, turning the palm backward.

"pseudo-CTS": A term coined by Ray Wunderlich, Jr., M.D., this refers to conditions which, although their symptoms mimic those of Carpal Tunnel Syndrome, have their origins in any of a wide variety of other disorders.

repetitive strain injury: In reference to the wrist, when the wrists or hands are used repeatedly over long periods of time, the muscles and tendons become susceptible to microscopic tearing and fatigue. Without sufficient rest and time to heal, chronic inflammation results, leading to redness, heat, or swelling, and pain from inflamed nerve endings.

rheumatologists: These doctors are specialists in disorders of the joints, muscles and associated structures, such as arthritis, degenerative joint disease, and myositis (inflammation of muscle tissue).

subluxations: Misalignments of the spine which cause nerve irritation.

supination: Referring to the hand, turning the palm forward.tendinitis: Inflammation of the tendons. Also spelled **tendonitis.**

tendons: Tough bands of connective tissue that attach muscles to bones.

TENS: A small, battery-operated device wired to electrode patches attached to the patient's skin, the TENS unit uses electrical pulses which seem to stimulate the body's own natural painkillers. Also known as **transcutaneous electrical nerve stimulation.**

ultrasound: Used for therapeutic purposes, ultrasound uses high-frequency sound waves to increase blood flow to an injured area, to warm muscles, to relieve pain, and reduce tissue inflammation and edema.

vertebrae: The 33 bony segments of the spine.

Workers' Compensation: An insurance program mandated by federal and states governments requiring employers to cover lost wages and medical expenses for employees who are injured on the job.

Overuse Injury Checklist

Use this check list to keep a record of your symptoms. It can also be helpful to share with your physician when you go for an examination. Make copies of this page to document your progress as you go through treatment.

1) **PAIN**   0=no pain 10=worst pain
   Fingers L _____ R _____ (which fingers?) _____
   Hand L _____ R _____
   Wrist L _____ R _____
   Forearm L _____ R _____
   Shoulder L _____ R _____
   Shoulder Blade L _____ R _____
   Neck L _____ R _____

2) **NUMBNESS**   1=never 2=occasionally 3=most of the time 4=constant
   Fingers L _____ R _____ (which fingers?) _____
   Hand L _____ R _____
   Wrist L _____ R _____
   Forearm L _____ R _____
   Shoulder L _____ R _____

Shoulder Blade L _____ R _____

Neck L _____ R _____

3) **TINGLING**   1=never 2=occasionally 3=most of the time 4=constant

Fingers L _____ R _____ (which fingers?) _____

Hand L _____ R _____

Wrist L _____ R _____

Forearm L _____ R _____

Shoulder L _____ R _____

Shoulder Blade L _____ R _____

Neck L _____ R _____

4) **WEAKNESS**   1=never 2=occasionally 3=most of the time 4=constant

Fingers L _____ R _____ (which fingers?) _____

Hand L _____ R _____

Wrist L _____ R _____

Forearm L _____ R _____

Shoulder L _____ R _____

Shoulder Blade L _____ R _____

Neck L _____ R _____

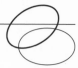

Resources: Where to Go for Help

Organizations

American Physical Therapy Association
1111 No. Fairfax St.
Alexandria, VA 22314

The Arthritis Foundation
800-283-7800

Feldenkrais Resources
P.O. Box 2067
Berkeley, CA 94702
510-540-7600

Fibromyalgia Network
5700 Stockdale Hwy. #100
Bakersfield, CA 93309
805-631-1950
(Newsletter, doctor referrals, booklets)

The Job Accommodation Network is listed in the RSI @BP:Newsletter as a service of the President's Committee on Employment of People with Disabilities, operating out of West Virginia University,. It offers a toll-free information service to people in the U.S. and Canada who need information about specific work-related situations. Their toll-free number is 800-JAN-7234.

Labor Occupational Health Program
University of California at Berkeley, School of Public Health
Berkeley, CA 94720
510-642-5507
(Catalog of publications, videos, training materials)

**The National Arthritis and Musculoskeletal
and Skin Diseases Information Clearinghouse**
Box AMS
Bethesda, MD 20892
301-495-4484

National Institute of Neurological Disorders and Stroke
Office of Scientific and Health Reports
Building 31, Room 8A16
Bethesda, MD 20892
301-496-5751
(Information on cumulative trauma and computer-related injuries)

National Institute of Occupational Safety and Health
Mail Stop C19
4676 Columbia Parkway
Cincinnati, OH 45226
800-356-4674
(Information on workplace safety)

Onsight Technology Education Services (Gary Karp)
1510 Eddy Street, Suite 1511
San Francisco, CA 94115
415-749-1983
(Wide range of ergonomic products, training and evaluation services)

Reflex Sympathetic Disorder Association
P.O. Box 821
Haddonfield, NJ 08033
(RSD resources)

Electronic Resources

If you have access to a computer, a modem, you can tap into the wealth of information available through the Internet and the World Wide Web. You can find thousands of resources throughout the world simply by entering a "Search" for any of the topics covered in this book. RSI's, ergonomics, natural medicine, Workers' Compensation—literally anything you might be looking for is available.

The computer world is constantly changing, and although these electronic addresses were correct at the time of publication of this book, I cannot guarantee their accuracy in the long term. **The Repetitive Strain Injury (RSI) Electronic Newsletter** is a must-have for those of you with access to the Internet. Free of charge to electronic subscribers, the bimonthly *RSI Newsletter* is full of up-to-the-minute information on products, publications, support groups, and includes articles from experts in the field as well as from patients around the world. Subscription is easy. Simply send an E-mail message to:
    <majordomo@world.std.com>.
Leave the subject heading blank. Send the message: SUBSCRIBE RSI. That's it.

SOREHAND: SOREHAND is an international discussion group/bulletin board also accessible through the Internet. To subscribe to SOREHAND, send an E-mail to this LISTSERV address:
    <LISTSERV@UCSFVM.UCSF.EDU>.
Leave the subject heading blank, then send this message: SUBSCRIBE SOREHAND your name. SOREHAND is a bit trickier to get—your request will be answered with a confusing message asking for confirmation within 48 hours. It took me four tries to successfully sign on, but it's worth the trouble.

Dan Wallach provides a helpful resource for people looking for information about typing injuries, including reviews of keyboards, software tools, and furniture. The Typing Injury Archive is available via anonymous ftp:
    ftp://ftp.csua.berkeley.edu/pub/typing-injury

Typing Injury FAQ (Frequently Asked Questions) can be accessed in a subdirectory there:

   ftp://ftp/csua.berkeley.edu/pub/typing-injury/typing-injury-faq

And everything can be found from Dan's World Wide Web page:

   http://www.cs.princeton.edu/grad/dwallach/tifaq

Books

Ergonomics, Work and Health by Stephen Pheasant (Macmillan, 1991).

Healthy Computing: Risks and Remedies Every Computer User Needs to Know by Dr. Ronald Harwin and Colin Haynes (Amacom, 1992).

Listen to Your Pain by Ben E. Benjamin (Penguin, 1984).

Living Yoga by Georg Feuerstein and Stephen Bodian (Jeremy P. Tarcher, Inc., 1993)

The Natural Treatment of Carpal Tunnel Syndrome by Ray C. Wunderlich, Jr., M.D. (Keats Publishing, Inc., 1993)

Relaxercise, by Mark Reese and David Zemach-Bersin. Available from Feldenkrais Resources 800-765-1907.

Sitting on the Job (How to Survive the Stresses of Sitting Down to Work—A Practical Handbook) by Scott Donkin (Houghton Mifflin, 1986, 1989).

Soft Tissue Pain and Disability (2nd ed.) by Dr. Rene Cailliet (F.A. Davis Co., 1988).

Available from North Coast Medical, 800-831-9319, order #NC74501, but must be ordered by a health professional.

Stretch and Strengthen by Judy Alter (Houghton Mifflin, 1986).

Sugar and Your Health by Ray C. Wunderlich, Jr., M.D., Good Health Publications (Johnny Reads, Inc., 1982).

Treat Your Own Neck, and *Treat Your Own Back* both by Robin McKenzie (Spinal Publications New Zealand, Ltd).

Also available from North Coast Medical, order #NC89009 and NC89008, respectively.

Workers' Compensation Claims by Gwen Hampton. For ordering info, call 818-247-8224.

Yoga, the Iyengar Way by Mira, Silva and Shyam Mehta (Alfred A. Knopf, Inc., 1990)

Articles and References

"Biomagnetic Arthritis Treatment," *The New York Times* (January 17, 1993) LI section, p. 8.

"Brachial Plexus Tension Tests and the Pathoanatomical Origin of Arm Pain," Elvey R.L. (1979)

In: Glasgow E.F., Twomey, L., *Aspects of Manipulative Therapy* (Melbourne: Lincoln Institute of Health Sciences, 1979) 105-110.

"Double crush syndrome: Cervical radiculopathy and carpal tunnel syndrome," Osterman, Pfeffer, Chu, et al. Presented at a meeting of The American Society for Surgery of the Hand, New Orleans, LA, 1986

"Cure Carpal Tunnel Without Surgery: A $3 Bottle of Vitamin B6 May Be

All it Takes," *Natural Health* magazine (July/August 1993) pp. 63-64.

"The Double Crush in Nerve Entrapment Syndromes," Upton A.R.M, A.J. McComas, *The Lancet* (August 18, 1973) 2:359-361.

"Entrapment Neuropathies of the Upper Extremities," David M. Dawson, *New England Journal of Medicine* (December 31, 1993) 329 (27) 2013-2018.

"Keyboard Induced RSI," *The New York Times* (March 2, 1992, Science Times section) pp. B5-B6.

"Medical Magnetism—A Healing Force Coming of Age," by Martin Zucker, *Let's Live* magazine, March 1993

"Neck Muscles Play Part in Carpal Tunnel Syndrome," Pronsati, Michelle P. *Advance for Physical Therapists* (July 6, 1992).

"Overuse Syndromes of the Upper Extremity in Interpreters for the Deaf,"Cohn, L., Lowry, R.M., Hart, S., *Orthopedics* (February 13, 1990) (2):207-209

Karr I.M., *Osteopathic Medicine* (Acton MA, Publication Sciences Group. 1975) pp. 183-199.

"The Relationship of the Double Crush to Carpal Tunnel Syndrome: An Analysis of 1,000 Cases of Carpal Tunnel Syndrome," L. Hurst et al, *Journal of Hand Surgery* 10B(2):202-204, 1985.

"A Review of Physical Exercises Recommended for VDT Operators," K. Lee, et al, *Applied Ergonomics,* Volume 23, No. 6, pp. 387-408, 1992.

"Role of B6 Examined in Carpal Tunnel Syndrome," D. Goldberg, *The Chiropractic Journal* (August 1987).

"Shoppers' Guide to Input Devices," in *Computer Shopper* (August 1993) pp. 262-270; chart, pp. 273-282; company phone numbers, p. 282.

"Symptoms May Return After Carpal Tunnel Surgery," *The Journal of the American Medical Association* (April 17, 1991) 28, 8:674

"Treatment of Arm Pain Associated With Abnormal Brachial Plexus Tension," Elvey R.L., *Australian Journal of Physiotherapy* 32 (4)1986.

"The Upper Limb Tension Test—the S.L.R. of the Arm," Kenneally, Rubenach, Elvey, in: Grant R, (ed)*Clinics in Physical Therapy: The Cervical and Thoracic Spine* (New York: Churchill Livingstone, 1988).

APPENDIX C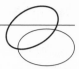

Product Information

As I worked on this book, it seemed everywhere I looked I found new devices and gadgets designed for RSI sufferers. I've tried to list some of them here, in the hopes that you'll be able to find something that will allow you to function more effectively. Check your own local medical supply companies, stores that specialize in natural foods or nutrition, computer supply distributers, drug stores—there are products out there that can help make your life easier, but it may take a bit of searching to find them. Here are some companies with products or catalogs to help you get started.

AbleNet
800-322-0956
(Adaptive devices for people with disabilities)

AliMed
97 High Street
Dedham, MA 02026
800-225-2610
(Catalog of ergonomic products, medical supplies)

American Ergonomics
100 Shoreline Highway
Building B, Suite 295
Mill Valley, CA 94941
415-388-2300
(chairs and other products)

Anabolic Laboratories
P.O. Box C19508
17802 Gillette Avenue
Irvine, CA 92713
714-863-0340
(Wrist splints, forearm braces, cervical pillows, and other orthopedic supplies)

Apple Computer Disability Solutions Store—Aisle 17
800-600-7808
800-755-0601 (TTY)
(Catalog of assistive technology products for the Macintosh user)

Biological Homeopathic Industries, Inc.
11600 Cochiti S.E.
Albuquerque, NM 87123
800-621-7644
(Traumeel ointment and tablets)

Body Wise™ International, Inc.
6350 Palomar Oaks Court, Suite A
Carlsbad, CA 92009

Conair Corporation
150 Milford Road
East Windsor, NJ 08520
800-3-CONAIR
(Sonassage Sonic Pain Reliever)

DeNikken, Inc.
Westwood Place, Suite 250
10866 Wilshire Blvd.
Los Angeles, CA 90024
(Biomagnetic products)

Direct Safety Company
7815 South 46th Street
Phoenix, AZ 85044
800-528-7405
(Industrial safety products)

Enrichments Catalog
Box 32
Brookfield, IL 60513
800-323-5547
(Products designed to make life easier for those
with difficulty lifting, gripping, etc.)

ErgoForm
800-452-3827
(Cold packs)

Ergosource
2828 Hedberg Drive
Minnetonka, MN 55343
800-969-4374
(Many ergonomic products, videos, and training materials)

Grab On™ Products
100 N. Avery Street
Walla Walla, WA 99362
1-800-8GRABON
(soft pen/pencil grippers)

Microcomputer Accessories
5405 Jandy Place/P.O. Box 66991
Los Angeles, CA 90066
1-800-521-8270
(Wrist Reminder™, Wrist Trolley™, many other products)

National Easter Seal Society
P.O. Box 06440
Chicago, IL 60606-0440
312-726-4258; fax: 312-726-4258

Making Life Better: Catalog of Catalogs—This catalog offers many products that are essential for children and adults with disabilities who seek to live their lives as independently as they can. The cost of the catalog is $5, prepaid. This includes postage and handling and a $5 bonus certificate toward the purchase of publications about disability awareness and prevention.

North Coast Medical, Inc.
(800) 821-9319
(Catalog of ergonomic products)

Smith & Nephew Rolyan Inc.
One Quality Drive, P.O. Box 1005
Germantown, WI 53022
(800) 558-8633
(Large informational catalog of ergonomic health and safety products)

Therapeutic Appliance Group
P.O. Box 339
Woonsocket, RI 02895-0781
800-457-5535
(Handeze Gloves)

Therapy Skill Builders
3830 E. Bellvue/P.O. Box 42050-Y
Tucson, AZ 85733
602-323-7500
(Rhino Grippers Hand Strengthening System)

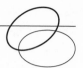

Index